Teaching Yoga for the Menstrual Cycle

of related interest

Menopause Yoga
A Holistic Guide to Supporting Women on their Menopause Journey
Petra Coveney
Foreword by Dr Louise Newson
ISBN 978 1 78775 889 6
eISBN 978 1 78775 890 2

Teaching Body Positive Yoga
A Guide to Inclusivity, Language and Props
Donna Noble
Foreword by Jivana Heyman
ISBN 978 1 78775 335 8
eISBN 978 1 78775 336 5

Hypermobility on the Yoga Mat
A Guide to Hypermobility-Aware Yoga Teaching and Practice
Jess Glenny
Foreword by Jules Mitchell
ISBN 978 1 78775 465 2
eISBN 978 1 78775 466 9

Teaching Yoga *for the* Menstrual Cycle

AN AYURVEDIC APPROACH

Anja Brierley Lange

Foreword by Dr Shijoe Mathew

SINGING DRAGON
LONDON AND PHILADELPHIA

First published in Great Britain in 2023 by Singing Dragon, an imprint of Jessica Kingsley Publishers
An imprint of Hodder & Stoughton Ltd
An Hachette Company

1

A CIP catalogue record for this title is available from the British Library and the Library of Congress

ISBN 978 1 83997 247 8
eISBN 978 1 83997 248 5

Printed and bound by CPI Group (UK) Ltd, Croydon, CR0 4YY

Jessica Kingsley Publishers' policy is to use papers that are natural, renewable and recyclable products and made from wood grown in sustainable forests. The logging and manufacturing processes are expected to conform to the environmental regulations of the country of origin.

Jessica Kingsley Publishers
Carmelite House
50 Victoria Embankment
London EC4Y 0DZ

www.singingdragon.com

Contents

Part 2: Anatomy and Physiology

Part 3: Teaching Cycle-Aware Yoga

Foreword

by Dr Shijoe Mathew

Practicing *Āyurvedic* medicine in the UK, occasionally I come across the concern that traditional medicines like *Āyurveda* are quite possibly outdated, and hence probably unsuitable for the ailments and lifestyle disorders we face in this modern era. Currently, we know quite a lot about how our body functions and have evidence-based remedies with reasonably positive outcomes. But as we go deeper into understanding, beyond specific anomalies within a hormone or structural issues with a joint into how these bodily systems interact with each other, how our mind and body interact with each other, how the nature, the sun, the moon, the seasons, etc. influence our physical and mental health, the modern scientific understanding is still in a developing state and evidence starts pointing towards the benefit of a holistic/multidisciplinary approach rather than a purely reductionist one.

Growing up in a village in the southern Indian state of Kerala, where the healthcare system is uniquely an amalgamation of modern acute healthcare facilities and traditional herbal medicine for everything else, it never occurred to me that healthcare is always an institutionalised affair. For me, the home remedies like herbal decoctions or oils that my mom prepared for common ailments gave the important feeling of knowledge accessibility when it comes to maintaining wellbeing. The values and customs, herbs and oils, scents and prayers imbibed into me growing up made me think; that being self-aware, nature awareness, and at the same time staying proactive with one's own physical and mental health needs were basic steps towards meaningful living. Studying *Āyurveda* for six years at university later reinforced these values, while developing scientific knowledge and clinical skills, but wasn't sufficient to prepare me for the role of a "translator" I would later have to be.

When my journey as a doctor in *Āyurvedic* medicine took me to the UK in 2016, little did I realize that my role here would have to be that of a specialized "translator"; not someone who translates language, but the philosophy of being! Here we are quite used to taking fast-acting remedies for everyday concerns like heartburn, headaches, and other digestion issues without paying much attention to the reason behind these symptoms. Subtle signs from the body like dryness, irregularities in menstrual cycles, sensitivities, discomfort, and intolerances are easily covered up or ignored until it is unmanageable using over-the-counter pills which is when we often take expert advice. On the other hand as an *Āyurvedic* doctor, nothing is more valuable than an opportunity for early intervention based on these early warning signs.

Health is a complex act of coordination; it's essentially balance or homeostasis. It's not just the coordination of physical and chemical entities, it is the entire act of living in tune with nature. Dividing the body into microsystems and managing their specific functions with precision has indeed improved our ability to recover from acute injuries and life-threatening disease conditions. But in the case of fine-tuning life, based on our body clock and its interaction with the environment, we need multiple perspectives leading to a wholesome picture. The superiority of this approach is especially evident with chronic inflammation and metabolic disorders, especially in their early state.

When Anja consulted me a few years back to understand how *Āyurvedic* herbs could help her with some of her own health concerns, I could sense the thirst for knowledge within her. With her experience of studying *Āyurveda* already in India and of course extensive yoga training, Anja was very aware of the principles behind *Āyurvedic* medicine and was a firm believer in its potential to help her. Little did I know at that time that she would be creating such a masterpiece, bringing together various perspectives of understanding menstrual health. Not only that, but being an experienced yoga teacher, she was beginning to create a toolbox that is extremely useful from a practice point of view.

Anja continued her yoga work with students during the COVID lockdown. I followed her posts online sharing valuable thoughts as well as nuggets of information regarding the pelvic organs, menstrual health, the *Āyurvedic* perspective of common women's health issues, yoga, etc. which I found a helpful resource to point to for my other patients who are not so proficient in *Āyurveda* yet. At that point, I thought it would be great to have a compilation of this information in one place.

Anja's book is brilliantly structured, paying attention to key details, starting from the ancient *Sāṅkhya* philosophy to recent research studies, respecting cultural values and being aware of differences associated with feminine anatomy, and physiology. The book explains the basic principles of *Āyurveda* and the Sanskrit language-based terminologies in a simplified and relatable manner, making it accessible for any readers who are from outside India and not familiar with either already. Through the explanations, it is very clear how *Āyurveda* and yoga are connected through their core philosophy, where the former specialises in therapeutics and the latter in setting the pathway to deeper mental and spiritual well-being.

I was fascinated to see the amount of background information Anja has gathered to support the texts, ranging from ancient Vedic period literature to British medical journals. The book also successfully brings together *Āyurvedic*, yogic as well as modern medical views to form a well-rounded understanding of menstrual health and wellbeing. The explanations seamlessly connect both the world revealing the beauty of her in-depth awareness in this field and her experience which finally reflects on the chapters detailing the practical applications.

The menstrual cycle and the hormonal changes associated with it are nature's clever way to facilitate a highly energy-consuming activity of gestation, into a more practical and sustainable system. The process of preparing the female body and mind for creating the most perfect environment to sustain a new life has to be precise with little room for error. From an *Āyurvedic* point of view, in every menstrual cycle, the whole of the uterine reproductive system undergoes a reset, and everything that remained unused in the last cycle is flushed out. *Āyurveda* considers this as a natural cleansing procedure that happens in a women's body regularly each month. The significance of this cleansing is not just on renewing the reproductive function, but it is on the entire body. In different stages of the hormonal cycle, *Āyurveda* understands the influence of different elements, especially the air and fire elements, and the cascading impact this has on the hormones, metabolism, skin, and mind. The book reminds us that we must be aware of various factors affecting hormones and shape our routine practice to facilitate a healthy transition, especially in the natural stages of hormonal change, to avoid any negative health impacts.

This book that Anja has created is a solution for the prominent barriers I faced while starting my *Āyurveda* practice in the UK. Specialists from different spheres of science with knowledge of *Āyurveda* will hopefully be inspired by this creation to further their knowledge and eventually share such incredible resources with mankind. I also hope that the readers of this book will feel empowered by the knowledge to challenge their current yogic practice and evolve their understanding of both yoga and *Āyurveda*, especially in the Western world, to make it further accessible to more and more people interested in it.

Although Anja has indicated that the level of information in this book is mainly for yoga teachers and practitioners, every woman in my view should be equipped with this knowledge to guide her choices and help deliver the optimum possibility of living life to the fullest. I shall end by wishing Anja the best on the occasion of such a magnificent milestone in her yogic life and hope it reaches millions of people, enlightening their pathway through the light of knowledge. I'm humbled, excited, and grateful for the opportunity to write a foreword for Anja's creation.

अज्ञानतमिरान्धस्य ज्ञानाञ्जनशलाकया ।
चक्षुरुन्मीलतिं येन तस्मै श्रीगुरवे नमः ॥

ajyaana timiraandhasya
Jnaana anjanashalaakayaa
chakshurunmiilitam yena tasmai shriigurave namah

Salutation to the teacher, who helps open the eyes blinded by darkness of
ignorance with the coryllium stick of knowledge

May we honour and embrace
Mother Nature's cycles and seasons
the phases of the moon
the tides of sea

the wisdom of our wombs

Introduction

The menstrual cycle is so much more than menstruation. The whole monthly cycle is a fascinating flow of changing hormones and *doṣas* (*Āyurvedic* physiology). As hormones and *doṣas* change, so will mood, energy and physiology. These are shifts half of the population will experience.

And, of course, this cycle will affect how we approach and experience our yoga practice.

Sometimes we, or our students, feel strong, motivated and powerful. The muscles grow and repair easily. And other times our coordination is off, we are fatigued and we easily overheat. Maybe there is more risk of injury or a sense of hypermobility.

These are natural fluctuations happening through the menstrual cycle. Yet, it is something daily life, society and most yoga practices don't acknowledge. *Āyurveda* recognizes these changes. *Āyurveda* provides a framework for how to live *with* the menstrual cycle, as well as the cycles of life and the seasons.

If you have a menstrual cycle, or your students do, then it's time to appreciate the powers of the different phases of the cycle. It's time to work *with* the cyclic nature rather than against it or ignore it. We need to understand how we can practise yoga to support the body, its changing phases and our emotional wellbeing.

Somehow this wisdom has been omitted from most yoga teacher training courses and biology lessons. And what we don't know, we don't know. In this book, you will learn *Āyurvedic* principles to apply to your yoga teaching and practice. You will be educated in the Western understanding of the cycle and how it affects us. You will understand menstrual cycle awareness from a Western and *Āyurvedic* perspective. Regardless of what style of yoga you teach or practise, you will have the foundation and knowledge to create yoga sessions based on the individual and their cyclic nature. You can apply this knowledge to general menstrual health, specific menstrual health complaints, if you teach womb yoga or fertility classes, the education of womb wisdom, or something completely different.

This book is intended for yoga teachers, to expand and enhance the knowledge you have from your trainings and practical experience. It aims to bring yoga, *Āyurveda* and menstrual cycle awareness together in a practical way. The information is also encouraging for yoga practitioners and those sharing *Āyurveda* through consultations. It is for those who menstruate and those who share their lives with them – perhaps as a yoga teacher. Maybe you have a great interest in yoga and *Āyurveda*; maybe you also offer red tents or Goddess/women's circles.

When I discovered *Āyurveda*, my yoga practice and teaching started to make complete sense. It was the missing piece of the puzzle. It is through my continuous study, practical application, lived experience and all the people who have come to class, private sessions, trainings and consultations that this book has evolved. I hope it will offer you a combination of yoga, Western science and *Āyurvedic* wisdom to inspire and enhance your own yoga journey, along with that of your students.

Menstrual cycle awareness

If you have a menstrual cycle, do you track it? I am curious, because for a long time I didn't. I would put a note in my diary when I got my period and then a sign 28 days later when, according to the 'textbooks', I would get my next period. Obviously, my periods weren't 28 days apart. They rarely are. Only 12.4 per cent of people have a 28-day cycle (Soumpasis, Grace & Johnson 2020).

But it's not all about menstruation. It is about all the shifts that happen in the body through the cycle, how the phases of the menstrual cycle affect the hormones, physiology as well as the mental and emotional state of being. From an *Āyurvedic* perspective, we also acknowledge these rhythms. This includes the fluctuating energies of the day, the lunar month, the seasons, our lifetime as well as the menstrual cycle and how it all relates to our unique constitution. Interestingly, menstrual cycle awareness is definitely gaining popularity. Some sports coaches and personal trainers now recognize how hormones can affect training, including recovery and muscle gain. It is a growing topic in popular literature and on social media.

As you read through the book you will understand both the Western science view and *Āyurvedic* knowledge and wisdom, and how to implement it into your yoga and your daily life.

HOW TO TRACK THE MENSTRUAL CYCLE

I suggest menstrual cycle tracking in the book because it is such an excellent compass and guidance. And it is very simple. Either get a journal or use an app where you make notes about how you feel through the month. Day 1 is the first day of the period and then it continues for however long the cycle is until the next period. I suggest keeping some kind of tracking continuously. You can jot down your energy levels, emotional state, appetite, if you feel strong, flexible or fatigued, if are you feeling assertive, outgoing or contemplative.

Once you notice a pattern, you can work with your cycle rather than simply ignoring it or even working against it. You will learn how as you read this book.

Use of Sanskrit language

The *Devanāgarī* alphabet is said to be the language of the Divine. It is the Sanskrit letters that in themselves can be *mantras*. I am not a Sanskrit scholar and my knowledge is very limited. However, I honour the original language used to convey both yoga and *Āyurveda*. I have relied heavily on the Wisdom Library website (www.wisdomlib.org) and Nicolai Bachman's *The Language of Āyurveda* (2006) and *The Language of Yoga* (2005) for the transliterations of Sanskrit words and terminology. Any mistakes, omissions and faults are entirely my own.

The Sanskrit transliterations are italicized and we have chosen that the specific topic of this book, *Āyurveda*, is capitalized throughout the book. Although it is not grammatically correct, I have pluralized some words such as *doṣas* and *cakras* – but not *āsana*. Certain words such as *cakra* are often written as *chakra* and *doṣa* as *dosha* in modern texts, but for consistency, I have tried to work with the classical transliterations.

Cultural appreciation and appropriation

When I first discovered yoga in the 1990s, there wasn't any debate about cultural appropriation, and I am still in the process of learning. I grew up in Denmark as a white person in a very white environment. My teachers were Danish too, and from the Satyananda School of yoga tradition. In a way, they were stereotypes of the 1970s and 80s yogis/yoginis in their orange clothes. I loved them and I fell in love with my yoga practice.

Most of my yoga teachers have been Western but not all. In India, I studied at the Sivananda Ashram where we had Indian teachers, among other nationalities. My teachers of *Āyurveda* at Middlesex University were Indian and Sri Lankan, having studied in their respective countries. I also had the pleasure of studying in India with Indian *Āyurvedic* doctors.

I loved India even before I went. I have spent months there both travelling and studying yoga as well as learning in *Āyurvedic* hospitals. Mother India and her people have a very special place in my heart. As a white Western woman, it is my intention that all I am sharing shows appreciation and respect for *Āyurveda* and yoga.

The feminine, the masculine, gender and sex

From an *Āyurvedic* perspective, we are all *Śiva* and *Śakti*, the masculine and the feminine, the God and the Goddess. We talk a bit about the concept of *Puruṣa* and *Prakṛti* in Chapter 2 on *Sāṅkhya* philosophy where *Puruṣa* is the supreme cosmic energy of *Śiva*, and *Prakṛti* the Divine Mother of *Śakti*.

In our manifest form, we may identify with either or neither gender.

The references and my own language refer to female anatomy and physiology, meaning the physical differences between the male and female sex rather than the gender one may identify with. This includes research such as 'female athletes' or 'women in sports'. As I am female, a woman, with a menstrual cycle I also express my own experiences. Writing from my passion and embodied experience, I include words such as I, we, us, our, as part of the flow of the book.

I acknowledge that you may or may not have a menstrual cycle for which there can be many reasons. You may be male with an interest in serving your menstruating students better. You may identify as female, male or non-binary or something completely different. This is not a book for one specific gender. All are welcome and appreciated.

How this book is arranged

This book is divided into three parts. Part 1 is the very foundation of this book. We explore the importance of menstrual cycle awareness. You will be introduced to *Āyurveda* in general and in the context of yoga as well as some of the important *Āyurvedic* terms used throughout the book. We look at cultural context, myths and wisdom.

In Part 2, we dive into the fascinating topic of anatomy, physiology and hormones from both a Western and *Āyurvedic* perspective, and we look at how it applies to yoga.

We get practical in Part 3, learning how to bring it all together. This includes teaching for each phase of the cycle as well as looking at yoga for common menstrual complaints. We explore the importance of rest and rejuvenation.

Enjoy the journey

This book has grown from the seeds planted along the way. Some seeds became blogs or social media posts and some encouraged further research, study and training as well as the teaching of fellow yoga teachers. Others evolved into workshops, teaching about menstrual cycle awareness through yoga classes, *Āyurvedic* discussion or a combination of both. Some seeds became my online course Feminine Cycles and Seasons (menstrual cycle awareness and *Āyurveda* for womb wellness). From this ever-evolving journey, the book emerged. I could keep writing, keep researching, adjusting and editing because life is fluid, things change and we are always learning.

If you are new to *Āyurveda* and menstrual cycle awareness you will receive an in-depth foundation as well as practical skills to incorporate these practices into your yoga classes.

Āyurvedic practitioners will be aware that there is much more to *Āyurveda* than what I share here, yet you will appreciate how to view yoga from an *Āyurveda* perspective.

Yoga and *Āyurveda* are for the individual, and a book cannot cover every single person's unique situation. Rather than being prescriptive, this book is for education and inspiration.

I am excited to share my knowledge with you and hope this book will be part of your continued growth and inspiration.

PART 1

BACKGROUND AND INTRODUCTION

CHAPTER 1

Yoga and the Menstrual Cycle

Why do we need *Āyurveda* and menstrual cycle awareness in yoga?

Just like there are yearly seasons, and the moon changes through the month, we are also cyclical beings. As humans, we have several cycles. The one we are most familiar with is the circadian rhythm, which is the 24-hour cycle of waking up in the morning, having breakfast, going to work, commuting home, eating dinner, resting and then going to bed at night. We follow this rhythm each day, except for weekends when we do the daily chores such as shopping and cleaning instead of going to work.

Our society and culture follow this linear rhythm as the only way to live. We expect to be the same, achieve the same, feel the same, be evenly creative and productive within this 24-hour cycle; disregarding where we are during the menstrual cycle, whether it is a warm summer day or we are in the midst of the dark cold winter. We have never learned that there is another way.

But we are also influenced by the infradian rhythms, which acknowledge the longer cycles, such as the yearly cycle, the seasons, the moon cycle and the menstrual cycle. However, most people are not aware of just how much the infradian rhythms influence us and these shifts are generally not taken into account in how we live our life.

We are conditioned to be and feel the same rather than appreciate our cyclic nature and hormonal changes. We are encouraged to be positive, energetic and 'nice' people, all the time. Most women grew up being told to be a 'nice girl'. This kind of gender stereotyping affects how we view the changing phases of the menstrual cycle. Women may strive (because of this kind of view) to be resourceful and take care of others. This is more natural in certain parts of the menstrual cycle. But in other parts of the cycle, such as in the premenstrual phase, we take the rose-tinted glasses off and come into our assertive focused self – a part that may not be appreciated by society and therefore ourselves.

The same goes for our yoga practice. We expect to continue the same routine and practise the same poses, with the same power and strength, even when our hormones and the *Āyurvedic* concept of the *doṣas* tells us to slow down or adjust our practice. Because that is how we have been conditioned and are expected to be. But we are cyclical, not linear. There are positives in all our phases: we just need to change our mindset. This is what menstrual cycle awareness and *Āyurveda* are about. In *Āyurveda*, this is what we do: be aware of our inner cycles as well as the external shifts and environmental seasons. It is time to harness the power of the changing phases of the menstrual cycle. Working *with* the body rather than *against* it. And that is where the principles of *Āyurveda* can guide us in life, through the menstrual cycle and in our yoga practice.

The yoga influence in the West[1]

This cyclical wisdom seems to have been lost in how we practise modern Western yoga in mainstream yoga studios and yoga classes. Considering that most current yoga practitioners in the West identify as women it is interesting how menstrual cycle awareness has been taken out of our yoga practice (Cartwright *et al.* 2020; Cramer *et al.* 2016; Yoga Journal and Yoga Alliance 2016). Perhaps it is because much of the yoga we practise today has been inspired by men – teachers with male anatomy and physiology and who don't have firsthand experience of the menstrual cycle.

Consider Krishnāmacharya. He is often thought of as the father of modern yoga. Born in 1888, he was the yoga teacher for renowned yogīs such as K. Pattabhi Jois, B.K.S. Iyengar, Srivatsa Rāmaswami, A.G. Mohan and his own son T.K.V. Desikachar. These are all male practitioners who have influenced contemporary yoga classes. However, he did have one female yoga student who became a very notable teacher in her own right, Indra Devi (1899–2002) (Tirumalai Krishnamacharya, About KYM).

There are many other teachers, but let's remind ourselves of a couple of these famous influential yogīs who trained under Krishnāmacharya.

K. Pattabhi Jois, of *Aṣṭāṅga Vinyāsa* yoga, was born in 1915. Although he didn't have any specific modifications for the menstruating body, the traditional Mysore style would close their *Shala* (yoga studio) during the full and

1 I have to highlight the allegations of abuse, sexual abuse, rape and cultism of some of these teachers, their senior teachers and the establishments around them. Please refer to Matthew Remski's tireless work and Uma Dinsmore-Tuli's Yoni Śakti: the Movement for further details, more education and support for those affected.

new moon. He also recommended a 'lady's holiday' for the first three days of menstruation (Ashtanga Yoga Austin). *Aṣṭāṅga Vinyāsa* yoga was part of the inspiration for many notable creative *vinyāsa* flow yoga styles such as Jivamukti yoga and Shiva Rea's *Prāṇa Vinyāsa* flow.

B.K.S. Iyengar influenced the alignment-based yoga practice. He was born in 1918. In his book *Light on Yoga*, he makes some references to 'menstrual disorders'. However, his alignment cues were the same for the male and female bodies (Iyengar 1991). His daughter Dr Geeta Iyengar has a greater influence on how to adapt her father's style of yoga to female physiology and anatomy and has written several books on this topic.

Another branch of modern yoga rose from Swami Sivananda's teachings. Swami Sivananda was born in 1887 in South India and practised as a physician before moving to Rishikesh to focus on his spiritual life, setting up an ashram and writing books on yoga, *Vedānta* and other spiritual topics (Swami Sivananda). Two of his disciples started popular styles of yoga that were my introduction to the practice and influenced me greatly.

One disciple was Swami Satyananda Saraswati, born in 1923, who founded the Satyananda style of yoga and the Bihar School of Yoga. My very first yoga classes were in this style and although I teach very differently, it is a style of yoga I have kept going back to as a student. The Bihar School of Yoga has published several books on various subjects of yoga, yoga philosophy and spirituality, probably the most famous book being the orange covered *Āsana Prāṇayāma Mudrā Bandha*, but it also published the *Nawa Yogini Tantra*, which is a book on yoga for women (Saraswati 1996).

The well-known Sivananda yoga style was founded by Sri Swami Vishnudevananda born in 1927. There are Sivananda centres across the globe sharing this style of yoga. I did my very first yoga teacher training with them and stayed in one of their ashrams in India for several months.

I don't recall any specific modifications or adjustments associated with the menstrual cycle, female physiology or anatomy while training with any of these styles of yoga. Certainly, the main influence of the yoga styles came from a male teacher, with a male anatomy and physiology perspective. It is as if the 'standard' is the male body. And although the female anatomy and physiology differ, we are still assumed to practise the same. This is not just in yoga, of course; this is historical and affects all aspects of life. Caroline Criado Perez writes in her book *Invisible Women* (2019), 'Seeing men as the human default is fundamental to the structure of the human society.' We see this repeated in medical research and sports science. This is a concern we will return to as you read through the book.

My point is that most of these people are male, and most of their students would most likely have been men as well. Not only would the generalized alignment cues be directed at mostly male students but rarely would it consider the menstrual cycle. We have two issues here. One is physical alignment and technique appropriate for the female anatomy which is different from the male. Another is how hormonal changes affect our body, mind, emotions and energy. Our changes are also doṣic (a combination of the five elements in our being). From an Āyurvedic perspective, and therefore also from a yogīc view, our energy and doṣic influence shift through the menstrual cycle. This is what we will focus on in this book.

Implementing our cyclic nature into our life and yoga

It is my intention that through reading this book you will gain greater insight into the wisdom and logic of *Āyurveda* and the *doṣas* so that you can apply it to your yoga practice and when teaching your students. *Āyurveda* is about living with nature, the seasons and the cycles. It's about getting to know what our body and energy need. It is working with nature rather than ignoring or working against it.

If we ignore these shifts and pretend the female physiology is like the male, we completely disregard the powers of each phase of the cycle. We work against the hormonal fluctuations and the *doṣic* changes. The male and female hormones and *doṣic* shifts are different. We have different phases and rhythms and so our yoga practice (and life in general) should reflect these important changes, working with our body and energy to embrace the power of our rhythms.

There is still a lack of research in the area of female physiology and how the menstrual cycle affects us in terms of medicine, surgery, general wellbeing and sport. It was only in 2016 that the US National Institutes of Health (NIH) 'implemented a policy requiring investigators to consider sex as a biological variable' (Woitowich *et al.* 2020). Before that, most research was conducted on a majority of male participants, completely ignoring how the female sex hormones and physiology might respond to treatments and how the different phases of the cycle could be a factor. A review by Liu and Mager (2016) states that researchers 'viewed women as confounding and more expensive test subjects because of their fluctuating hormone levels'. 'The perceived complexity and higher costs of studies if women are included' were other reasons for being excluded (Ravindran *et al.* 2020). To me, these are the exact reasons why we should explore and study the menstrual cycle. And the phases can have a positive influence in medical intervention; for example, one study about treatment for breast cancer showed that those 'operated on during the luteal phase had a significantly better prognosis than patients operated on during the follicular phase' (Veronesi *et al.* 1994). Our cycle matters.

We are seeing more research on female athletes in sports sciences. I will refer to some of this throughout the book. We may not think of yoga as a sport – and certainly, yoga as a spiritual practice is not a sport at all – but for most modern Western yoga classes we can use the research in sport sciences as a reference along with the ancient wisdom of *Āyurveda* and yoga. For example, some research suggests that women are more prone to ligament damage during certain phases of the cycle. There are phases in the cycle more conducive to building up muscle and strength too. In *Āyurveda*, we can compare this to how the qualities of the *doṣas* are increasing or decreasing during the cycle.

So why wouldn't we work with the cycles instead of ignoring them? In this book, I will reference Western research and how it compares to *Āyurvedic* wisdom, making it applicable to your yoga teaching and practice.

People in the sports and research sphere such as Stacy Simms and Kelly McNulty are both trailblazing, sharing and encouraging research into the female athlete, the menstrual cycle and how the hormonal changes affect us and our sports performance depending on where we are in the cycle. Yoga teachers such as Shiva Rea have influenced me, and many others, to embrace and include *Āyurveda*, the female energy and cyclic nature in my yoga practice and teaching. Uma Dinsmore-Tuli is another influential teacher sharing yoga for women's health.[2]

So let's start to consider our cyclic nature as we embrace our yoga practice or as we teach others. Let's ask how their cycle is encouraging them to notice how they feel during the month, how their energy is, their mood, strength, flexibility and determination. Then we can practise and align with their body rather than ask them to fit into a certain style or sequence of yoga. We can allow their body, hormones, *doṣas* and energy to guide the practice.

This is yoga. And *Āyurveda*. Connecting to our body, mind, heart and energy. Our body wisdom. Our womb wisdom.

---

2 Please note that Western research is relatively new compared to *Āyurveda*, discoveries are made continuously, and including and focusing on the female cycle and female athletes is even more recent. If you refer to any studies, it is always worth reading the whole study and making an effort to investigate more recent papers. At the time of writing the research I refer to is, in my opinion, valuable as a reference.

My introduction to yoga, *Āyurveda* and the menstrual cycle

When I did my yoga teacher training courses, no one mentioned the menstrual cycle. I was educated and trained in how to modify and adapt to common injuries or health concerns. I consider my basic 200 hours of training an excellent foundation for starting as a teacher. From there I was able to build on, grow and continue my education.

I did have a short introduction to *Āyurveda* as a sister science to yoga but there was not much on how to apply the principles to my yoga teaching or practice.

At the time of my training (1998 and again in 2005) – before social media, before period-positive communities on Instagram, hashtags and awareness campaigns – menstrual cycle awareness and even fertility yoga weren't really discussed. We didn't acknowledge how hormones and the *doṣas* change through the monthly cycle or how they affect us and our yoga practice. A basic yoga teacher training is just that: basic and a foundation. It is only when we start teaching that we understand the nuances, that one sequence, one style of alignment, flow, pace does not fit everybody. And that is where the real learning starts. You picked up this book to continue your education, to continue to learn. It is a never-ending journey.

When I became interested in *Āyurveda* and later studied it, I started to connect the dots. After a workshop with the renowned *Āyurvedic* doctor Robert Svoboda at the London Sivananda Yoga Centre, everything fell into place. I began to understand why an individual and seasonal approach to yoga makes a difference, and why people need different styles of yoga. The *Āyurvedic* principles made complete sense to me, to my daily life, my health and my yoga. It was then I decided to go to university as a mature student to study *Āyurveda* full time. I enrolled at Middlesex University for my Bachelor of Science degree and postgraduate degree. In the last year, we had apprenticeships in *Āyurvedic* hospitals in India, embracing the richness of *Āyurveda*, and the culture and energy of India.

I continued (and still do) my yoga training with Shiva Rea, who was the first teacher I saw blending the knowledge of yoga and *Āyurveda*. She also shared a more creative style of yoga, including yoga for female physiology and anatomy.

A short introduction to *Āyurveda*

If you are not familiar with *Āyurveda* I will give you a proper foundation soon, but for now, here is a short introduction.

Āyurveda is the traditional Indian medical system. It is still practised widely today in hospitals with highly qualified *Āyurvedic* doctors and surgeons.

Āyurveda is about the individual. The *Āyurvedic* system acknowledges that each person has a unique constitution and has unique experiences affecting their health and how they feel. This includes the seasonal changes, the time of day and so on. It also includes the changes through life: childhood, through adulthood to old age. *Āyurveda* appreciates the cyclic nature of female physiology.

Learning about *Āyurveda*, I understood that people who have a menstrual cycle also move through different phases during the month, just as Mother Nature moves through winter, spring, summer and autumn. And as the moon moves through the lunar cycle of the new moon, through the full moon to the dark moon.

In *Āyurveda*, we adapt our routine, diet and behaviour according to the seasonal changes, the weather and how we feel in our body and energy. In this way, we are in harmony with nature, and with ourselves.

It only makes sense that we would do the same with the menstrual cycle, adapting according to our cyclic nature.

We are changing through the menstrual cycle. The hormones change and fluctuate. From an *Āyurvedic* perspective, our *doṣas* shift. Here *doṣa* refers to an energy and its specific qualities, which we will get into later in the book.

If our *doṣas* and hormones change, why don't we start to work with those changes rather than ignoring them or, even worse, working against them?

If, in *Āyurveda*, we would consider changing our diet from cold salads in the summer to warm soups in winter, why wouldn't we consider noticing our cravings and needs during our monthly seasons?

Modern science, yoga and *Āyurveda*

As mentioned earlier, sports science is starting to be interested in the menstrual cycle and how it affects sports performance. Some sports coaches are tracking their athletes' menstrual cycles so they can factor them into their coaching and training. While there is not much high-quality research in this area, and many studies contradict each other, it is encouraging that sports science and Western science acknowledge that the menstrual cycle affects us.

So although yoga isn't necessarily a sport and there are many aspects to yoga aside from the *āsana* (yoga poses), I feel we can still use both modern science and current research as well as *Āyurvedic* knowledge to support our students and ourselves through our menstruating years.

We can work with nature and harness the power of each phase of the monthly cycle rather than simply ignoring the qualities the different parts of the cycle offer.

This is what I want to do with this book.

As I am a Western yoga teacher in the UK, I mostly teach *āsana* (posture) based practices. I teach yoga poses and shapes, I teach parts of *haṭha* yoga and include the various styles of flow or *vinyāsa* yoga. That is my background and my experience. However, whichever lineage you may have as a yoga teacher or movement instructor, I hope you can apply this wisdom to your teaching and private practice too.

In the classic yoga texts that I have read or studied, there isn't much about cyclic living, but there is in *Āyurvedic* texts. In *Āyurveda*, we look at our cyclic nature. And although I might refer to Western science and hormones, the interesting thing is that it very much relates to the *Āyurvedic* concepts. It is simply different languages or different words. Sometimes I use the *Āyurvedic* language around our physiology. And I will remind you of the connection to Western science and the Western terms of hormones and physiology too.

As *Āyurveda* and yoga are sister sciences, I feel it is absolutely appropriate to compare and connect them. I had been practising yoga for ten years before I started my full-time degree in *Āyurveda*, and it was through *Āyurveda* that my yoga truly started to make sense. *Āyurveda* offered me words, principles and concepts that made my yoga practice and teaching complete and whole. I hope it will inform and bring more depth and understanding to your personal yoga practice and your yoga teaching too.

CHAPTER 2

Sāṅkhya Philosophy

The sister sciences of yoga and *Āyurveda*

It is often said that yoga and *Āyurveda* are sister sciences. What does this mean?

For us, in the West, we might only know a little of the history, culture and deeper spiritual aspects of yoga, but I feel it's important to spend a bit of time on yogīc philosophy. Or rather, one aspect of yogīc and *Āyurvedic* philosophy.

Hinduism and Indian culture include the teachings of six specific philosophies or *Ṣaḍ-Darśana*. These are philosophies or spiritual paths rather than religions and are all generally accepted as part of Hinduism. Yet they vary and can be interpreted in many ways.

The *Ṣaḍ-Darśana* are *Sāṅkhya*, *Nyāya*, *Vaiśeṣika*, *Mīmāṃsa*, *Yoga* and *Vedānta*. We won't go into the details of these philosophies. That's a whole other range of books and studies. This is just a reminder for you to appreciate the background of yoga and *Āyurveda*. All of these philosophies have influenced *Āyurveda*. But we will focus on yoga and *Sāṅkhya*.

Here we refer to yoga as a philosophy, not a Westernised exercise class or physically based *āsana* (posture) practice. Traditionally, yoga is a way to realize the Divine or Truth. Dr David Frawley (Frawley 2004, p.5) says: 'Yoga is the spiritual aspect of *Āyurveda*, while *Āyurveda* is the therapeutic branch of yoga.' But even the classical *Āyurvedic* texts, such as the *Caraka-saṃhitā*, explore the Divine, the Soul and how the world manifested.

It is beyond the scope of this book to look deeply into the history of yoga and its evolution and changes through time, although there are many excellent resources on this topic you may want to explore.

You may already be familiar with some of the concepts below but I have found that *Sāṅkhya* philosophy is one of the topics that is easily forgotten once we finish our yoga teacher training and the focus shifts to *āsana*-based yoga classes. The reason I share it here is to give you the background for just how interwoven yoga and *Āyurveda* are. More specifically, it is the foundation for how we approach the practical application of *Āyurveda* in the yoga practice.

Introducing *Sāṅkhya*

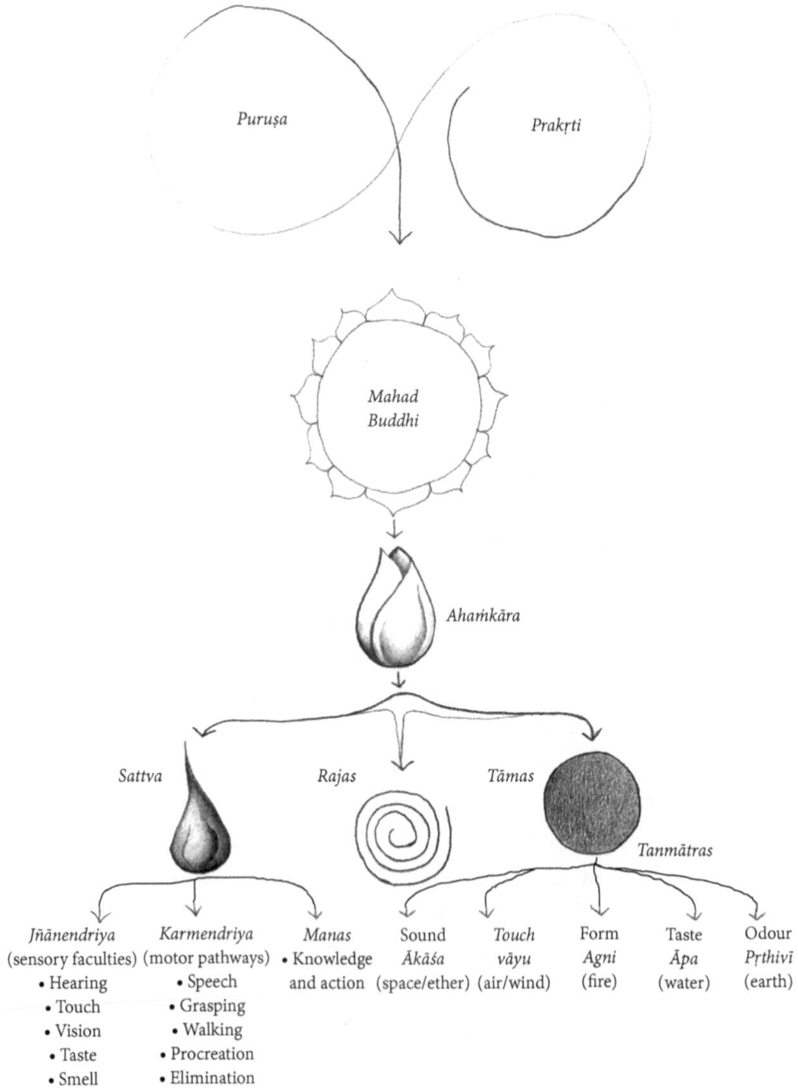

Sāṅkhya. The evolution from the unmanifest to the manifest

The word *Sāṅkhya* can be translated as *Sāṅ* meaning truth and *Khya* meaning realize. This philosophy is the foundation of the *Āyurvedic* principles as well as how many *yogīs* and *yoginīs* view the world – realizing the truth of life and the universe. *Sāṅkhya* can also be interpreted as systematic enumeration or related to numbers. It is this specific concept of numerations, or the 24 principles of *Sāṅkhya*, we will explore below.

Sāṅkhya philosophy is vast, deep and broad. I would highly recommend studying it if you enjoy yoga philosophy but this is by no means essential. To understand the principles and the practical application of yoga and *Āyurveda* for the menstrual cycle, we only need to know some of the concepts.

The 24 principles of Sāṅkhya philosophy

The enumerations of *Sāṅkhya* is an explanation of how the unmanifest becomes manifest. The unmanifest is the concept of *Puruṣa*. It is pure Consciousness and the Ultimate Truth. *Puruṣa* is formless and it is where it all begins. The 24 principles come into action when *Puruṣa* comes in contact with *Prakṛti*. This is the journey from Consciousness and the unmanifest to the manifestation of the physical – such as you and me.

Further in this book, we will focus on the last five principles in depth. These are the five great elements that form the practical application of yoga and *Āyurveda* during the menstrual cycle – and beyond. Most of the principles are commonly introduced in yoga philosophy and yoga teacher training courses.

1. *PRAKṚTI*

Prakṛti is the creative potential. It creates through the Consciousness of *Puruṣa*. *Āyurvedic* doctor Vasant Lad (2002, p.6) says, '*Prakṛti* is creativity, the feminine energy. Within the womb of *Prakṛti*, the whole universe is born. Therefore, *Prakṛti* is the Divine Mother.'

Prakṛti has another meaning as well. When we discuss *Āyurveda* later in the book it refers to a person's constitution.

2. *MAHAD*

When *Prakṛti* and *Puruṣa* come together, self-awareness manifests. This is *Mahad*. It is supreme intelligence and order.

3. *BUDDHI/AHAṀKĀRA*

Whereas *Mahad* is universal, it becomes *Buddhi* which is more individual awareness due to *Ahaṁkāra*. *Ahaṁkāra* can be interpreted as the feeling of 'I am' and our ego. Through *Ahaṁkāra*, the three tendencies or *guṇas* evolve.

THE THREE *GUṆAS*

Through the play between *Puruṣa* and *Prakṛti* and the movement of *prāṇa* (lifeforce energy) the *guṇas* of *sattva*, *rajas* and *tāmas* occur. It is through the three *guṇas* the rest of the principles manifest.

Sattva is often translated as pure awareness and equilibrium. *Rajas* is the energy of movement. *Tāmas* is inertia.

From a yogīc perspective, we aim for serenity and a harmonious *sattvic* nature. That is what our spiritual practice teaches us. When we are *sattvic*, we know when to activate *rajas* to pursue change, have the energy to get out of bed, enjoy our activities, work and so on. And we know when we need to employ *tāmas* to slow down, to rest and sleep.

Rajas can lead to agitation, selfishness and restlessness. *Tāmas* can also be lethargy, obstruction and ignorance. *Sattva* is the balance between *rajas* and *tāmas*.

The three *guṇas* influence the next principle of *manas* or the mind.

4. *MANAS*

Manas is sometimes translated as the mind. This is our faculty of processing the information we receive from our five senses: hearing, touch, vision, taste and smell. And these are what comes next in the evolution from Consciousness to matter.

The five *jñānendriya* or sensory faculties are:

- Hearing
- Touch
- Vision
- Taste
- Smell

Now we reach the concept of *karmendriya*, or the motor pathways, which we may also know from yoga:

- Speech
- Grasping
- Walking
- Procreation
- Elimination

As we move closer and closer in our manifested journey of matter we reach the objects of sensory perception or the concept of *tanmātras*:

- Sound
- Touch
- Form
- Taste
- Odour

Finally, we reach the five great elements; the *pañcāmahābhūtas*. These are the concepts we will explore much more in-depth in our journey of *Āyurveda*. The five elements are the basis of the *doṣas* and how we explore what happens in the menstrual cycle and how we approach our yoga practice and poses:

- Space or ether: *ākāśa*
- Air: *vāyu*. We will explore this specific element and its movements in greater detail later in the book.
- Fire: *agni*
- Water: *jala/āpas*
- Earth: *pṛthivī/bhūmī*

In a very simplistic way, *Sāṅkhya* philosophy reminds us that the 24 principles are the manifestations and interplay with *Puruṣa* or Pure Consciousness. We are *Puruṣa* but we identify with the physical and mental manifestation of the 24 principles. And it is through these manifestations we experience life.

There is much more to it than that, of course!

For now, remember the five elements as these are the foundations of our practical application of *Āyurveda* and yoga for the menstrual cycle. It is always good to remember the three *guṇas* of *sattva*, *rajas* and *tāmas* too, for our intentions in our yoga teaching or practice.

Prāṇa the lifeforce energy

Another aspect both yoga and *Āyurveda* have in common is the concept of *prāṇa*. *Prāṇa* is often translated as the lifeforce energy. It is the vital force. *Prāṇa* is difficult to translate and explain. We can say it is what brings life to existence. When we exhale the last breath, when the *prāṇa* leaves the body, we pass on, we die. *Prāṇa* is energy. It governs our body, our mind and our energetic being.

A disturbance in *prāṇa* disturbs the five manifested elements of space, air, fire, water and earth, therefore our *doṣas* and our physical, mental, emotional and spiritual wellbeing.

Many yogīc practices involve manipulating or encouraging a balanced flow of *prāṇa*. You may have heard that there is a connection between *prāṇa* and oxygen. *Prāṇa* isn't the oxygen but the vital force that makes oxygen or energy to support the body. *Prāṇa* is in our food and beverages, in anything living.

Consider the energy or *prāṇa* of junk food – food that has been manufactured in a factory, flown across the world, frozen and defrosted. Or perhaps tinned food. Reheated in a microwave oven. Perhaps of a slaughtered animal long dead before you finally consume it in front of the television. Then consider a farm-to-table meal, made out of freshly grown organic vegetables straight from the earth. Cooked with love in a happy environment. Eaten in the company of loved ones. What nourishes you? What is full of *prāṇa*?

Through our yoga practice, we can manipulate or encourage a healthy flow of *prāṇa*. In *Āyurveda*, we consider the movement of *prāṇa* in our physical and energetic body. We will go into the details of the movement of *prāṇa* in the section on the five great elements, or the *pañcāmahābhūta*, in Chapter 3.

CHAPTER 3

Understanding *Āyurveda* and the *Doṣas*

Āyurveda: An introduction

Āyurveda is the traditional Indian medicinal system. *Āyurvedic* doctors and surgeons have high university degrees comparable with Western medical education. In India, *Āyurveda* isn't an 'alternative' therapy. It is something people use for serious illnesses, for surgery as well as for general wellbeing, just like you and I may go to our general practitioner or hospital. The name *Āyurveda* can be translated as knowledge or science (*veda*) of life (*ayus*). *Āyurveda* isn't just about finding medication for an ailment but is a way to live in harmony to prevent dis-ease, to be in balance with life, nature and your true being. In the Hindu pantheon, Lord Dhanvantari is the god of *Āyurveda* and an avatar of Lord Viṣṇu.

Āyurveda has eight branches of medicine: internal medicine (*kāyachikitsā*), paediatrics (*bālachikitsā*), demonology or treatment of idiopathic disorders as well as psychiatry (*grahachikitsā*), ears, nose and throat (*śālākyatantra*), toxicity (*viṣacikitsā*), rejuvenation (*rasāyana*) and aphrodisiacs (*vājīkaraṇa*). In *Āyurvedic* hospitals, you will find consultants and departments specializing in each of these subjects as well as having more general practitioners.

Āyurveda can be traced from the ancient *Vedic* culture and sacred *Vedic* texts (classic Indian philosophy) and was originally an oral tradition. It is believed to be between 3000 and 5000 years old. The first written text on *Āyurveda* is thought to be the *Caraka-saṃhitā*, estimated to be from around 400–200 BCE. The *Suśruta-saṃhitā*, which is the main text exploring surgery in *Āyurveda*, is thought to be from the 6th century BCE. The third classical book in *Āyurveda* is the *Aṣṭāṅga-hṛdayam*. This treatise is estimated to have been compiled in 400 CE (Dick 2021; Loukas *et al.* 2010). These are the texts that inform the principles on all aspects of *Āyurveda* and the texts I keep referring back to. But there are also many newer more accessible books you can peruse to learn more about this science and philosophy.

Āyurvedic science is alive and continues to evolve. There are plenty of current research papers on *Āyurveda*, *Āyurvedic* treatments and medicines. It is a living science.

Āyurveda isn't just about diet, herbal medicine or body treatments. It is a way of life and a way to prevent imbalance to avoid illness. It has its spiritual component too, as we saw in the previous chapter introducing *Sāṅkhya* philosophy, and which is evident in the classic texts such as the *Caraka-saṃhitā*.

Our focus for this book is a holistic view of gynaecology (referred to as *prasūti* and *strīroga* in *Āyurveda*) as applied by yoga teachers and yoga practitioners to general wellbeing during the menstrual cycle. We will look at the menstrual cycle through the lens of *Āyurveda* and learn how to apply these principles to our yoga classes and practice in general.

The five great elements or the *pañcāmahābhūta*

We introduced the five elements as part of *Sāṅkhya* philosophy. Now we will fully explore each element in an *Āyurvedic* context.

THE FIVE GREAT ELEMENTS AND THEIR QUALITIES

Space or ether, *ākāśa*: all-pervading, expansive, holds everything; clear, light, subtle.

Air, *vāyu*: movement, dry, light, cold, rough, subtle.

Fire, *agni*: digesting, metabolic actions; hot, sharp, light, dry, subtle.

Water, *āpa*, *jala*: cool, fluid, dull, soft, oily.

Earth, *pṛthivī*: heavy, dull, dense, hard, cool.

Each of us is a unique combination of these five elements, which manifests as three *doṣas*. The three *doṣas* influence the menstrual cycle.

As we saw in *Sāṅkhya* philosophy, the elements manifest first with space, then air, followed by fire which creates water and finally earth. Let's look at the elements in detail. I am including the Sanskrit names as these are often referred to both in yoga and *Āyurveda*.

Space/ether/ākāśa

Ākāśa is spacious and all-pervading. The *guṇas*, or qualities, associated with *ākāśa* are clear, light, subtle, soft and immeasurable. *Ākāśa* can be light and spacious yet also ungrounded. It is where everything is manifested. We can not see it, although it holds everything.

We have space in our wombs. It obviously changes through our cycle but you may have heard the uterus is a hollow organ. I don't know if I agree with that statement but certainly, after birth it makes sense. For example, in *Āyurveda*, the postpartum period is an extremely special and important time. After birth, there is excess space where the element of air can move and potentially cause imbalance and therefore health concerns. This is why the fourth trimester, the 40 or so days after birth, is a time to be grounded, warm, oiled up, and nourished – basically, everything to prevent there being too much space and air elements!

Ākāśa is present in other parts of our being too, not just physically but also mentally, emotionally and energetically. Sometimes the elements are in perfect balance and sometimes there may be excess and imbalanced manifestations of the different elements.

Going back to the *Sāṅkhya* philosophy, *ākāśa* is connected with the *tanmātra* of sound and the *karmendriya* of speech.

In yoga, we consider the *ājñā cakra*, or the third eye, to be associated with the element of space.

Air/wind/vāyu

This is about movement and mobility. It is light, cold, dry, rough, subtle and can be erratic. We might not be able to see air but we can feel it on the skin. We can observe the effect of the air element as the wind blows.

The *tanmātra* is touch and the *karmendriya* are the hands or grasping.

The *viśuddhi*, throat, *cakra* has a connection with the element and movement of air.

This element is of importance to us as yoga teachers and as people aware of the menstrual cycle. In *Āyurveda* and yoga, we consider five subdivisions of the element of air or *vāyu*. These are also the five *subdoṣas* or subtypes of *vāta doṣa*. I will use the Sanskrit term *vāyu* to describe the subdivisions. Each division is connected with the breath and the movement of *prāṇa* in our physical and energetic bodies.

PRĀṆA VĀYU

It's our inhale and the meaning is the 'forward moving breath'. It is taking in the breath and letting it fill us up. It is also about receiving: food, nutrients, air and sense impressions. In yoga, we often associate *prāṇa vāyu* with the breath in general or an awareness we connect with in meditation and for spiritual evolution. The primary site is the head, although it is not restricted to this specific area.

VYĀNA VĀYU

This is the all-pervading movement of *prāṇa*. It's the outward moving air from our centre to our periphery. Often associated with the heart, it circulates energy to our whole being.

UDĀNA VĀYU

This is the upward moving flow of air. Think of it as the exhale, speech and coughing. It is associated with the diaphragm towards the throat. It is the force that helps us stand tall.

SĀMANA VĀYU

This equalizing breath is associated with the abdomen. It's a balancing movement of *vāyu* and supports our digestion.

APĀNA VĀYU

You will hear a lot about *apāna vāyu* in this book. *Apāna* is the downward movement of *vāyu*. Down and out. It's the exhale and the letting go. It's grounding us. It is responsible for elimination and reproduction. It initiates bowel movements, urination, ejaculation, childbirth and, of course, menstruation. *Apāna vāyu*'s seat is in the pelvis and the colon. Any obstructed or imbalanced *apāna vāyu* will affect the menstrual cycle. And actually, it will affect our overall health if we don't create harmony. The obstruction, excess flow or imbalance of *apāna vāyu* will affect the other *vāyus*, *doṣas* and our general wellbeing.

As we start to explore the menstrual cycle and yoga poses, we will come back to *apāna vāyu* and how we can support a healthy balanced movement of *vāyu* in the pelvic area.

Understanding how *apāna vāyu* is part of the menstrual cycle and the flow outward and downwards, of elimination and release, is important in working with the menstrual cycle. When we start to look at issues around menstrual health, we can perhaps see patterns with imbalances of the movement of *prāṇa* or the wind element.

As you can see, the wind element, specifically *apāna vāyu* and *sāmana vāyu*, influences our digestion too. Everything is connected.

Fire/agni

The fire of transformation and digestion. We not only digest our food but we also digest all our sense impressions. Every experience is an event that needs to be digested so we can take what is nourishing, learn the lessons from the experience and then eliminate what we no longer need.

Agni is one of the main pillars of health. We have several *agnis* but the one often discussed is *jāṭharāgni*, the digestive fire. If you go to an *Āyurvedic* practitioner or doctor they will most likely ask a lot about your digestion and bowel movements. Our digestion gives us great insight into our general health and wellbeing. In the *Caraka-saṃhitā*, it says that 'Strength, health, longevity and vital breath are dependent upon the power of digestion including metabolism. When supplied with fuel in the form of food and drinks, this power of digestion is sustained; it dwindles when deprived of it.'

The qualities of fire include being hot, sharp, light, dry and subtle.

The *tanmātra* is sight or vision and the *karmendriya* are the feet and walking.

The fire is the radiance and power of the *maṇipūra*, or navel, *cakra*.

Water/āpa/jala

This is fluidity in all its forms, not just water: the synovial fluid in our joints, the wetness of our eyes, the saliva in our mouth and so on.

The qualities of water are cool, liquid, dull, soft, oily and slimy. There are many variations of this flowing element in our body, in our mind and emotions, as well as in the external world.

The fluidity of water is often thought to be connected to our emotions, as well as to the tides, and therefore the phases of the moon as she pulls on the oceans.

The *tanmatra* of the water element is taste. Without water, there is no saliva and no taste. Since taste is something we want to enjoy, we also associate this with pleasure and sensuality. Perhaps unsurprisingly, the *karmendriya* is procreation and the reproductive system.

It is also connected with the *svādhiṣṭhāna cakra* or sacral energy.

Although we will focus on the elements and the *doṣas* in this book, you may find associations with how you can connect with the energetics of this *cakra* when you practise and teach yoga for the menstrual cycle.

Earth/pṛthivī/bhūmī

The element of earth is solid and stable. We can see and touch it. It has form and shape. The earth element grounds us. It has gravity and density.

The qualities of earth are heavy, dull, static, dense, hard and gross. It is 'building'.

The *tanmātra* is the sense of smell and the *karmendriya* is the anus or excretory organs.

As the element of earth is connected to the *mūlādhāra*, or root, *cakra* it also has a strong connection to the subject in this book. You may find that you bring in ideas and inspiration from your knowledge of the *mūlādhāra cakra* when you work with the pelvis and cycle.

Everything is a combination of the elements

We are all a combination of these five elements. Everything is. Some are lighter and more subtle than others. Some things are solid and heavy. A feather is light and airy. A big rock is dense and heavy. One is more air and space, the other more abundant in the earth element.

In a yoga class or yoga practice, consider the same qualities. A class can be based on each element to increase or balance some of those qualities. You may already teach classes around the elements.

As we move on to the menstrual cycle and the *doṣas*, we will see how each element, expressed through the *doṣas*, affects the different phases of the cycle, and how we can rebalance any potential imbalances appropriately.

Understanding the three *doṣas*

The five elements combine and create everything. Our body as well as our mental and emotional states are unique combinations of the elements. In *Āyurveda*, we group them into three functional principles called the *doṣas*. *Doṣa* is difficult to translate. The literal meaning is *fault* or *mistake*. But that's not how we generally talk about the *doṣas*. It is only when the *doṣas* come out of balance, vitiate, get misplaced or similar that they become a 'mistake'. But when in balance, the *doṣas* are principles or functions in our body and mind.

We, as human beings, will have a unique combination of the *doṣas*. The food we eat, the seasons, even our life cycle and menstrual cycle are influenced by the *doṣas*. We will get into how the menstrual cycle is affected by the *doṣas* in a little while. First, we need a short introduction to how the *doṣas* operate.

Let's look at the composition and function of the *doṣas*, starting with the five elements.

Ākāśa (space) and *vāyu* (air) become *vāta doṣa*.

Agni (fire) and *āpa* (water) are *pitta doṣa*.

Āpa (water) and *pṛthivī* (earth) are called *kapha doṣa*.

Knowing the properties of the five elements we already have an idea of the qualities of each of the three *doṣas*.

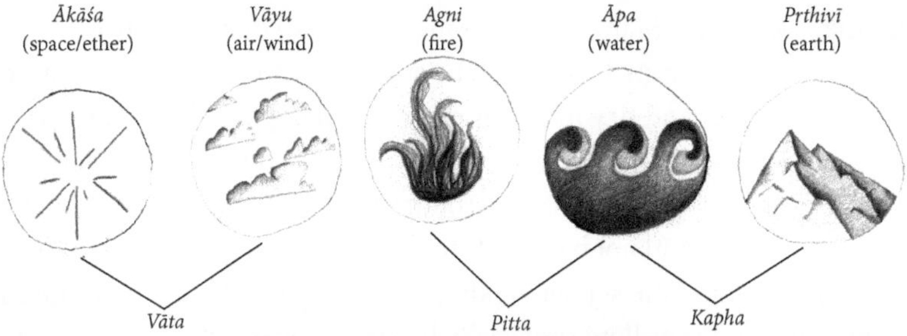

The five elements and the three doṣas

We say there are specific attributes connected with the three *doṣas*:

- *Vāta*: dry, light, cold, rough, subtle, mobile, clear.
- *Pitta*: hot, sharp, light, liquid, mobile, oily.
- *Kapha*: heavy, slow/dull, cold, oily, liquid, smooth/slimy, dense, soft, static, sticky, hard, gross.

How does this manifest in the *doṣas*?

VĀTA DOṢA

With the air and space element, *vāta* is light and breezy. *Vāta* is mobile. This can be actual movements such as fidgeting or the creative expression of dancing. It is also the movement of thoughts in our minds. These can be creative and inspiring, or they can create excessive movement causing anxiety and insomnia.

People influenced by *vāta* generally have a great imagination and like change. This can give rise to both fearfulness and feeling ungrounded. Physically, they tend to feel cold and dry.

As *vāta* is partly the element of wind it also carries the properties of all the *vāyus*, including *apāna vāyu*. This is the downward movement of wind responsible for elimination and menstruation.

This means that during the menstrual phase the body is influenced by *vāta doṣa* or, more specifically, *apāna vāyu*. In this context, *apāna vāyu* is doing its natural function. However, we may have blocked, imbalanced or excess *vāta* or *apāna vāyu*, in which case we need to restore balance. We can see an *Āyurvedic* practitioner but through our yoga practice, we can also start to work with the *doṣas* and our cyclic nature to maintain and find equilibrium.

Some individuals have more *vāta* in their constitution, because that's the way they were born. Many of us have increased *vāta* due to lifestyle.

Vāta-aggravating qualities are all the ones we mentioned in the box above. Eating light, cold and dry food, for example. Being in a dry, rough desert also increases *vāta*, as can the autumnal winds and shifts in weather. But for most of us, it's our lifestyle of lack of routine which vitiates *vāta doṣa*. Having constant thoughts and not being able to switch off. Being online, continuous scrolling, watching the screen, talking excessively and trying to multitask. Commuting and travelling (especially by air) increase *vāta doṣa*. Worrying increases *vāta* and is also a *vāta* quality.

We pacify *vāta* by reducing such activities, and by embracing warming, grounding, nurturing practices, routines and foods.

PITTA DOṢA

We often think of *pitta* as the fire element, although it is also water. Fire metabolizes, creates change and transformation. The light of the fire gives us a sharp clear vision. *Pitta* gets things done and has ambition. It makes quick decisions, sometimes without thinking of how an indecisive *vāta* person or a *kapha* friend who likes to take their time will respond to their idea.

Pitta people have the typical type-A personality. In excess, it's more human-doing than human-being. Doing too much and burning the candle at both ends can lead to burnout. Too much fire.

Pitta-aggravating qualities include hot, spicy foods and alcohol. Even hot power yoga.

Excess *pitta* can lead to increased heat such as heartburn, rashes and inflammation. It can manifest as anger, irritability, impatience and being short-tempered.

Because the *pitta* qualities are often celebrated in our society, many of us have excess *pitta*. It can be important to understand that there is a time to celebrate *pitta* and also a time to relax, cool and calm down a bit.

In the menstrual cycle, *pitta* is the spark that initiates ovulation. It is influencing the later part of the cycle, the luteal phase, where it helps metabolize the endometrium, or uterine lining, so it can be released during menstruation. If you feel the *pitta* fire of anger and irritability during the premenstrual phase, you may have a little (or a lot of) excess *pitta* in your system. Many perimenopausal symptoms such as irritation, hot flushes and dryness can be a build-up of *pitta doṣa*.

People with excess *pitta* benefit from learning how to cool and calm down, to take rest and appreciate doing nothing.

KAPHA DOṢA

This is the element of water and earth. These two elements are the densest, heaviest and most stable. A healthy *kapha doṣa* is grounded, has stamina and structure. Think of a Mother Earth-type goddess with big eyes and curves, full of love, devotion and calmness.

You can have too much of a good thing. When excess *kapha* becomes too heavy and too slow, it causes congestion. The body and mind can't metabolize properly and we become sluggish – both physically and mentally. Instead of love and compassion, we turn to greed, possessiveness and jealousy. Feeling low or depressed can also be manifestations of increased *kapha*. *Kapha doṣa* increases when we are inactive, not moving or exercising. If we don't use our brains, we encourage excess *kapha*. *Kapha* also increases if we eat too much cold, oily, heavy and dense foods.

But *kapha* people have stamina and strength. Encouraging dynamic movement like flow yoga, *vinyāsa* and breathing exercises is a great way to balance *kapha*.

In the menstrual cycle, the follicular phase is influenced by *kapha*. *Kapha* builds up the endometrium, or the uterine lining, after menstruation, creating a juicy, stable environment in the womb. It is the sensuous fertile flow of ovulation.

> You may want to bookmark this page if the *doṣas* are new to you. We will refer back to them again through the book and add more information and insights to these body-mind functions.

The individual unique constitution and the doṣas

Now we know a bit about the *doṣas* as concepts we can apply them to us as individuals, our life cycle and the menstrual cycle.

When we are conceived we are a unique expression of the five elements and the three *doṣas*. No one is exactly like us. We are unique. This is worth remembering when we teach yoga. No one is the same. We are all completely unique with individual constitutions, which in *Āyurveda* is called *prakṛti*. This specific expression of the *doṣas* may alter slightly while we are in the womb of our mother. When we are born, we have our *prakṛti*, our constitution. We discussed *prakṛti* in the *Sāṅkhya* philosophy section. Here it relates to us as individuals. We might have a lot of *vāta*, quite a bit of *pitta* but less *kapha*. Or something completely different. Our *prakṛti* is our uniquely balanced state of being.

Life, experiences, where we live, our diet, work, how we respond to stress, trauma, surgery, personal stuff, illness and so on affect our *doṣas*. For most of us, life will affect our constitution or *prakṛti*. Whatever we appear to be right now with all these changes is our *vikṛti*. Finding balance is not to have *vāta*, *pitta* and *kapha* even. It is coming home to our *prakṛti*.

> *Prakṛti*: The unique balanced combination of *doṣas* we had when we were conceived.
>
> *Vikṛti*: The current state of the *doṣas* and how they express themselves at this moment.

Even our life cycle from birth to death will be influenced by the *doṣas*. Childhood has more *kapha* as we build up and grow. Adulthood is more *pitta* as we need the power, ambition and focus to earn money, create a job and maybe a family (however that may look for you). As we grow older, we are influenced by the lightness of *vāta* as we don't need to engage the same way in the worldly sense but can focus on spiritual aspirations and the eventual letting go of life.

Wherever we are in life, as well as our constitution, will affect the menstrual cycle. Although this book is about the general shift of the *doṣas* in the menstrual cycle, note that this will affect us all differently because we are all unique beings with different constitutions, different experiences, coming from various cultures and beliefs.

Āyurveda is about learning to listen to our own body and understand when it's balanced and when we move out of balance. We start to become aware of how the environment affects us and we adjust to create balance.

For example, if we have a lot of *pitta* we avoid being out in the sun at midday. We might *want* to go to a hot power *vinyāsa* yoga class but we know it will add fuel to the fire so we enjoy a cooling *yin* practice or a slow flow instead. We eat less spicy or hot food.

In someone with a tendency to increased *vāta*, we try to avoid too much stimulation from social media and internet scrolling. We want to keep some kind of routine to stay grounded. To balance the coolness, lightness and airiness of *vāta* we eat warming foods like soups and casseroles. In our yoga, we may enjoy the creative *vinyāsa* flow yoga yet we focus on being steady, grounded and stable. *Yin* yoga to calm the mind is also excellent. A windy cold autumn day can increase *vāta* in everyone.

Feeling low and depressed may be from excess *kapha*. Dark, damp, cold winter days can increase *kapha doṣa*. So we remember to keep moving and breathing deeply or may add some dynamic breathing like *kapālabhāti* (skull-shining breath) or *bhastrikā* (bellows breath) *prāṇayāma*. *Vinyāsa* and any dynamic flow will keep us strong as well as offer us movement, flow and lightness.

Prāṇa, *tejas* and *ojas*

Associated with the three *doṣas* we also have the more subtle energies of *prāṇa*, *tejas* and *ojas*. As a yoga teacher, you have most likely heard about *prāṇa* and we mentioned it earlier in the introduction to *Sāṅkhya* philosophy.

Prāṇa

On a pure, undisturbed level, we can associate *prāṇa* with *vāta doṣa*. We have already discussed the movement of *prāṇa* as *vāyu* in our being. Although *prāṇa* is not the breath, one of its functions is respiration. Yet *prāṇa* is also what governs our biological functions, what lifts our soul and our mind. It is as light and all-pervasive as ether or space.

In yoga, *prāṇayāma* is a way to bring awareness to our breathing, our respiration and ultimately the movement of *prāṇa* in our being. There are practices to manipulate, lengthen and change the breathing patterns and therefore the flow of *prāṇa*. Some meditation techniques also manipulate or essentially enhance our *prāṇa*.

Tejas

Tejas is the pure fire of *pitta doṣa*. It is the illuminating light from the sun and the sacred fire, or *agni*. It is insight, clarity, knowledge and intelligence. We say we shouldn't play with fire. Too much, and the fire will burn and destroy. Excess hot yoga, heating and stimulating *āsana* or yoga flows may cause an imbalance in our *tejas*. It can burn us out, or we lose our luminous healthy glow, our inner light. Learning to listen to our inner wisdom and our body's intelligence will support our *tejas*.

Even gazing at a candle flame, such as in *trāṭak* meditation (candle gazing), enhances *tejas*. Walking in the sun and embracing sun salutations and solar energy practices with enlightened intelligence can help balance *tejas*, as does the understanding of the natural rhythm of sunrise and sunset.

Ojas

Ojas is the pure essence of *kapha* and the cool fluid watery element. *Ojas* needs a whole section on its own and we will discuss it further in Chapter 13 on rest and rejuvenation. But for now, we will keep it short and sweet. And sweet is what *ojas* is, like nectar, honey or ghee (clarified butter often used in Indian cooking and part of *Āyurvedic* medicine). *Ojas* is our immunity and vitality. It is the pure essence of *soma*, which is sometimes translated as bliss and is thought of as a plant or elixir of immortality. If we were to compare *Ojas* with Western science some would say it has the mood-balancing happiness and wellbeing action of the hormone serotonin.

We increase *ojas* with nourishing *sattvic* foods and activities. Pure love, *bhakti*, devotion and meditation may also improve *ojas*. Maybe a devotional or meditative yoga session can do the same with such an intention.

Ojas decreases when we are ill, when we take food, substances, beverages or activities that deplete or malnourish us. Experiencing trauma and stress decreases *ojas*. Excess exercise is depleting. This includes a very vigorous heating dynamic yoga session or breathing practices, particularly in hot spaces.

Sex, especially ejaculation, is also *ojas* depleting. *Āyurvedic* texts suggest that we can have more sex in the winter but less in the summer as hot summers can be depleting where we need more movement and heat in the cold winters. The stronger *kapha* types can be active with a good amount of sexual activities and while the lighter *vāta* people may love erotic fantasies, they get depleted more easily. *Pittas* are somewhere in between. However, lovemaking, which generates tenderness, love and the bonding hormone oxytocin, may help to increase *ojas*.

Finding subtle equilibrium

Just like our *doṣas*, we need balance and equilibrium between *prāṇa*, *tejas* and *ojas*. One supports the others. Too much *tejas* can burn out the *ojas*. *Ojas* depends on a healthy digestive fire, or *agni*, and so also on the more subtle *tejas*. *Prāṇa* depends on *ojas* to protect and support. It is a symbiotic relationship we need to care for.

You don't need to be an *Āyurvedic* practitioner or *Āyurvedic* doctor to apply these principles. We can encourage our students (and ourselves) to listen and check in on what is best for them (us) at that specific time. We can teach the same class to a room full of different people but allow them to adjust, modify and focus their attention on their own individual intention for the class and their individual wellbeing.

The challenge is knowing when we are listening to our ego or inner critic and when we are truly listening to our body, energy and inner wisdom. But that is exactly why we practise yoga. Learning to listen to our truth – not the ego!

When we have taught yoga for a while, we learn to listen to and read bodies. In smaller groups or private one-to-one sessions, we can ask questions and get to know our students. We can remind them when they might be listening to the ego rather than their body-wisdom and their energy; when to back off, or ease into the pose with more curiosity. We can encourage going a bit deeper with more intention. But in the end, it's their body. And no one knows their own body as well as themselves.

CHAPTER 4

The *Āyurvedic* and Cultural View of the Menstrual Cycle

Āyurvedic wisdom was for a long time an oral tradition. You will find many traditional *Vaidyas*, doctors, medicine men, women and elders who may very well have read the classical texts but have gained their healing wisdom from oral traditions. From father or mother to son and daughter. It's a living tradition. The classical texts, interpretations, commentary and translations were written in a time of patriarchal culture which may have influenced the tone of intended wisdom. Yet, we can still embrace the principles of *Āyurveda* and see its true wisdom as we meditate on and study the texts.

Āyurvedic gynaecology

The classical *Āyurvedic* texts such as the *Caraka-saṃhitā*, *Aṣṭāṅga-hṛdayam* and *Suśruta-saṃhitā* all have chapters on gynaecology and obstetrics and discuss menstrual health. They were very specific about the characteristics of healthy menstruation. We can find verses in the classic texts on various gynaecological complications and how to treat them.

According to the classics, healthy menstruation should appear every month after the age of 12 years and until 50. The colour is red as a hare's blood or of gunja fruits or a lotus. The colour may depend on the person's constitution. It should be easy to clean and have no foul odour. The *Vaidyas*, *Āyurvedic* sages, continue to discuss how the period should be five nights long, free from pain and neither excessive nor scanty.

The *Āyurvedic* doctors definitely found the monthly cycle an important part of health and wellbeing, much like we now are starting to recognize the menstrual cycle as the fifth vital sign, along with body temperature, pulse rate, respiration rate and blood pressure (ACOG 2015).

The strong focus on the menstrual cycle in the classical texts has partly to do with establishing a healthy pregnancy to get healthy children. At the time the texts were written, this was an extremely important aspect of culture, survival and family life. Having a family to support the family business, farmland, the elders and legacy was vital.

The texts further talk about sexual relations, sex positions, what time of the cycle is best for intercourse and when not to have sex. They advise not to have intercourse during menstruation but wait until after the bleed and until the 12th night of the cycle as that is a potential time of fertility. This is exactly as we advise today, with the understanding of ovulation and the survival of sperm within the female reproductive organs.

Sadly, I haven't found any beautiful poetry of living in sync with the menstrual cycle and honouring the bleed in the traditional *Āyurvedic* texts, much as I would have loved to. Instead, we find such interpretation in other spiritual texts and newer books on *Āyurveda*. For example, in the *Ratishastra*, thought to be written between 830 and 960 CE (Kokkoka 1965), it says, 'A woman who adorns her forehead with a mark made from Rochana mixed with the discharge of her own menstruation, is able to sway the whole world.' The *Yoni Tantra* (likely composed before the 11th century) pays homage to menstrual fluids as, 'Having seen the yoni full of menses, after bathing and reciting the *mantra* 108 times, a person becomes a Siva on earth.' There is power in menstruation.

Cultural context, myths and wisdom

The actual cultural context of yoga and *Āyurveda* is a vast study, so multilayered and specialized that it is beyond the scope of this book and my knowledge. Nevertheless, some of the myths, traditions and ideas may be worth looking into.

It is often thought that Indian culture suggests that menstruation is dirty. There are statements about not being allowed to cook because one is impure when menstruating, or you can't go to the temple because of being unclean. Indeed, some of the comments in the classical *Āyurvedic* texts also use the word 'unclean' in the translated editions.

But is being 'unclean' the actual reason for this?

From an *Āyurvedic* perspective, menstruation is indeed powerful. We have already discussed the five elements, the *doṣas* and the specific downward direction of *prāṇa* called *apāna vāyu*, the *prāṇa* or *vāyu* responsible for menstruation. It's a potent source of energy. From a more energetic or spiritual perspective, we can consider the idea of *kuṇḍalinī Śakti*. *Śakti* is a mover, with power and energy. *Śakti* is the creative force that makes things happen. *Kuṇḍalinī Śakti* is said to be the 'coiled power' or 'sleeping serpent' at the base of the spine waiting to be awakened. When *apāna vāyu* and *Śakti* are facilitating menstruation, it should not be interfered with. The energy is for the potency of menstruation.

Looking from such a perspective the reason for not cooking is not because of being unclean when menstruating. It is because *Śakti* and *prāṇa* are focused on the bleed through *apāna vāyu* rather than focused on the nourishment of the food. Perhaps it's not because of being impure that menstruating people are not allowed to visit the temples but because *Śakti* is already so powerfully present that it would be disrupting to their energy – and even that of others or the energy of the temple itself. Sinu Joseph (2020) quotes her Guru Pūjya Śrī Amritānanda Nātha Saraswathi, saying that, 'She [a menstruating woman] was so pure, that she was worshipped as a Goddess. The reason for not having a woman go into a temple is precisely this. She is a living Goddess at that time.' She further describes how some temples act on specific *cakras* as well as *apāna vāyu*, which 'could result in heavy bleeding or other menstrual disturbances' if one visits the temple during the menstrual phase.

Our spiritual practice is often more focused on the upward movement of *prāṇa vāyu* (such as in certain meditations) and while bleeding, the energy is governed by *apāna vāyu*, the downward force. This is what should be focused on and allowed to happen during menstruation.

We will discuss what impure or unclean means from an *Āyurvedic* perspective when we explore *Āyurvedic* physiology, but I want to introduce it here as it is understood from a practical and physiological *Āyurvedic* perspective.

Unclean, toxic and āma

In *Āyurveda*, there is a concept called *āma*, which is often translated as toxins or toxic. It really means undigested material, which can become toxic. Toxic means it is detrimental to our health. It's different from toxaemia or being poisoned. It also has nothing to do with modern clean-living or the detox fads we often see here in the West. This undigested material can be from food and beverages; it can also be excess or imbalanced *doṣas* or undigested thoughts, emotions and experiences. If we have any imbalances or excess of anything they have to go somewhere. Often the first place we will experience *āma* is in our digestion. It can also manifest as congestion in our minds. And it can go to our tissues (in *Āyurveda* we have seven *dhātus* or bodily tissues) or other body parts. One such tissue is *rakta dhātu*, or the blood. So if we have any excess *doṣa* or perhaps *rajasic* energy (anger, frustration, irritation) it can manifest in the menstrual blood. It is not that we are unclean or impure, as we might translate as dirty in the West. It is simply something in excess or imbalanced. In our spiritual practice, we certainly don't want too much *rajas;* rather, we favour a more *sattvic* energy.

In other cultures and religions, we see similar patterns as in the Indian culture. For example, in some Jewish traditions, *niddah* (menstruation) is seen as impure. A similar view is seen in both Christianity, Catholicism and Islam. Women are requested to retreat during their bleed and not perform spiritual practices, and clean themselves in a ceremonial bath after menses (Sridhar 2019).

As cultures, religions and politics are intertwined and for most of the world these have been completely influenced by patriarchy it is sadly easy to see how menstruation and generally women's bodies have been viewed as 'different' and therefore inferior and impure. As recently as 1878 the *British Medical Journal* published several letters discussing whether or not menstruating women could cause meat to become rancid.

Menstruation, the actual bleed, can be a powerful, energetic time. We can also allow it to be a spiritual practice of retreating, contemplation and simply being, or as Nithin Sridhar (2019, p.49) says, 'the whole process is considered as highly sacred and purifying in nature, which sets women free from Karmic bondage'.

Contemplations for you as an individual and as a yoga teacher

What is the attitude to the menstrual cycle where you grew up, live now and where you teach yoga? Consider your own thoughts when talking about the cycle in your yoga classes. How do you discuss this with your one-to-one clients? Or do you not mention it at all? If you have a menstrual cycle, how was your own experience of menarche (your very first period)? What did you know about the monthly cycle? Even if you are not a menstruating person, are you educated in the monthly hormonal changes?

These are important questions because we don't know what we don't know. Many of us weren't taught much in school or by our parents. And unless you have a special interest you might not look into the menstrual cycle at all.

It's only recently that we have started to talk openly about periods. Perhaps thanks to Instagram where there has been a bit of a revolution when it comes to sharing about menstrual cycle awareness and where menstrual cups, reusable or organic pads and tampons are advertised and where we see selfies of influencers in period pants. Now we talk about menstrual products rather than sanitary or hygiene products. Adverts no longer have blue rather than red fluid representing menstrual blood. Things are changing.

But it's not long ago that we refrained from physical exercise classes in school because we had our period. Not because it was painful, just because that's what we did. We hid our tampons when going to the bathroom. We only whispered about our cycles and certainly wouldn't mention it to our exercise or yoga teacher. The terms 'female trouble' and 'women's issues' were an excuse not to do certain activities yet also a way of not having to engage with what that actually meant.

The bleed was 'a curse'.

I don't remember much from my sex education or biology lessons on the menstrual cycle in school. It would have been helpful to understand more about our cycle, how the hormonal changes affect us and how we can embrace each phase. It feels a bit as if our whole cycle was reduced to the fact that menstruation was simply a sign telling us we weren't pregnant; it was bypassing all the other incredible things happening throughout the cycle.

There is still much education to do, more to learn and explore. What I find interesting is that perhaps patriarchy used the word 'unclean' or created taboos around the menstrual cycle and specifically the period. But before that happened and in the culture of yoga and *Āyurveda*, the menstruating person was full of *Śakti*, of energy and power, and therefore highly influenced by and influencing others, including spiritual places and energy in general. And that the menstrual phase was a way to naturally release *āma*, as we will discuss later. Menstruation wasn't taboo or dirty. It was a period of power and great spiritual insight.

CHAPTER 5

Lunar Flow and Connecting with the Moon

The moon phases and the lunar calendar

The word menstruation is interestingly the same in many languages, or certainly very similar. It derives from the Latin *mensis*, meaning month. This word comes from the Greek *mene*, translated as the moon. The menstrual cycle in *Āyurveda* is called *ṛtucakra*. *Rtu* means season and *cakra* can be translated as cycle or wheel, referring to a season or cycle such as the moon cycle.

There is no doubt we always felt a connection between the menstrual cycle and the actual moon cycle. Many people speak of the menstrual cycle as the lunar cycle or moon cycle. 'I am on my moon' is another way of saying 'I'm on my period'.

The actual moon cycle is around 29.5 days. The 'textbook' menstrual cycle is said to average 28 days, but for most people, it is either a little shorter or longer.

Is it a coincidence that the menstrual cycle is the same length as the lunar cycle? Maybe. Most of the world uses the Gregorian calendar of the 12 months which form a solar year, the time it takes for the earth to move through our seasons and around the sun. But before that, we adhered to the lunar cycles, something many cultures and religions still do.

According to the lunar cycle, the month is one whole lunation. This is the time from the new moon, through the waxing moon, to the full moon, then the waning moon to the dark moon. And so the lunar cycle starts again.

Many Indian festivals and celebrations are according to the lunar cycle, as is Ramadan and other Muslim holidays. We see this in the Jewish and Chinese calendar too. But it does not just feature in religious traditions. Folklore uses the phases of the moon. And if we look at biodynamic farming, we use the phases of the moon to understand when to sow the seeds and when to harvest.

Anecdotally you may have heard that emergency rooms in hospitals are busier on the full moon, and the police are attending more fights and disorderly behaviour. I can't find any hard facts or evidence for these claims. But just knowing we had a calendar and timed our tasks with the moon phases is interesting. We know the moon pulls on the sea and the tides. Would it be so strange if the moon affected us too? After all, we are sensitive to light and we are also mostly made out of water. Could the moon pull on our cycles, tides and emotions too?

The menstrual cycle, the moon and the doṣas

In *Āyurveda*, we find that the menstrual cycle, the *doṣas* and the moon are very similar. Let's start with the new moon. New beginnings, new month. This would be associated with day 1 of the menstrual cycle. The day we start our bleed.

Then the moon slowly starts to wax, or grow, onto the darkness of the sky, as the endometrium, or uterine lining, grows in the womb. It builds up. This is similar to *kapha doṣa*, the qualities of building, nourishing and cooling energies.

The apex of the lunar month is the full moon. The full moon is glowing, abundant, bright and mesmerising, just like the juiciness of *kapha doṣa*. And like ovulation.

Now the moon starts to wane, getting smaller in the sky, preparing to let go. This is the *pitta* time in the menstrual cycle or the luteal phase.

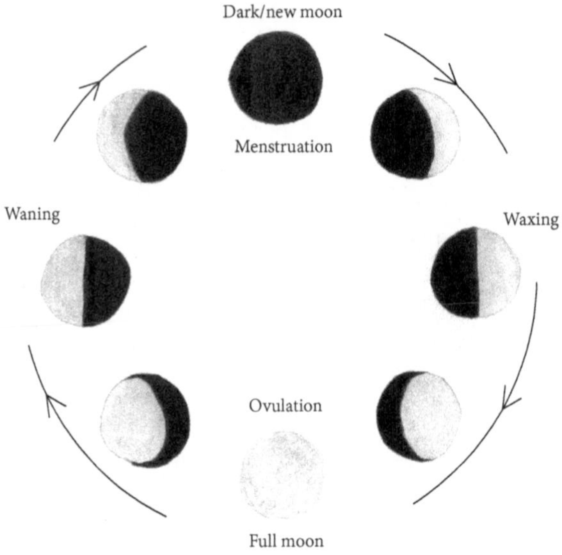

The phases of the moon cycle

For some *Āyurvedic Vaidyas*, this would be the perfect scenario. In her *Vedic* teachings, Maya Tiwari (Mayatitananda 2007) discusses the importance of connecting the menstrual cycle back to the moon for healing, both as a physical practice and perhaps more so on a spiritual level. In reality, most menstruating people shift between bleeding on the full moon, then mid lunar cycle, moving to the new moon and back again. Or perhaps you are always menstruating on the full moon or a waxing moon.

I am aware that other traditions have different opinions on what it means when we bleed at different times in the moon cycle but either way don't get too obsessed with how you may or may not align. Just notice how your cycle and the lunar cycle connect.

What I do love about this association is that if we do not have a menstrual cycle we can still connect with the moon cycle. So if you find the information in this book interesting or work with the moon but do not have a cycle then use the information above to connect your yoga practice or teachings with the actual moon.

Our students and clients may not have a menstrual cycle for many reasons. Perhaps they have amenorrhea (no menstruation) due to low body fat/body weight or RED-S (relative energy deficiency in sport), perhaps they are on medication, had a hysterectomy, have polycystic ovary syndrome (PCOS), are postmenopausal – perhaps they are on contraception or hormones. Trans and non-binary people may not have a period but have a sense of a cycle too. Due to medication, transgender women could still have symptoms of premenstrual syndrome (PMS) even if they don't have a period.

Regardless of having a cycle or not, we must listen to the needs our body and energy at any given time.

PART 2

ANATOMY AND PHYSIOLOGY

CHAPTER 6

Anatomy Awareness

Structures and organs

Everything is connected.

I say this a lot in my yoga classes and training courses – because it is true. Understanding our anatomy and physiology is a vast subject. As yoga teachers, we don't need to know everything but a few things are really useful and interesting to understand. Let's start with a bit of anatomy relating to the menstrual cycle.

Our pelvic bowl holds our pelvic organs. If you put your hands on your hips, or ask the average person to do so, we usually place the hands on top of the pelvic bones. This is the iliac crest. We have the 'hip points' at the front, which are our anterior superior iliac spines (ASIS). If we slide the hands further down we arrive at our hip joints. This is the place where the head of the femur inserts into the hip socket. These are towards the groin. The greater trochanter of the femur, or thigh bone, is the widest part of what we commonly call the hips. Now the fingers meet very low at the pubic bone, or rather pubis bones, connected by strong ligaments at the front. If you slide the fingers underneath your buttocks you'll find the sitting bones or ischial tuberosities. If you put the hands back on the iliac crests (commonly the hips) and slide them back you'll find the sacrum. The sacrum is the flat triangular bone just at the top of the buttocks. It is connected to the ilium via the sacroiliac joints. At the end of the sacrum, we have the tailbone or coccyx.

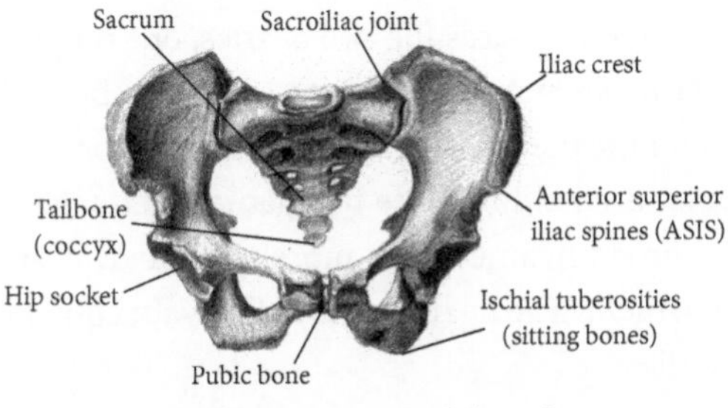

The bone structure of the pelvis

That's the pelvic bowl or the bony structure of the pelvis. Regarding the menstrual cycle, what's interesting is what's inside the pelvis. We will refer to the 'textbook' female pelvis.

Place the index fingers just above the pubic bones, palms of the hands touching the lower belly with the thumbs together forming a downward-facing triangle. This is sometimes called *yoni mudrā*. Your index fingers are approximately near the site of the uterus. And little fingers near the ovaries.

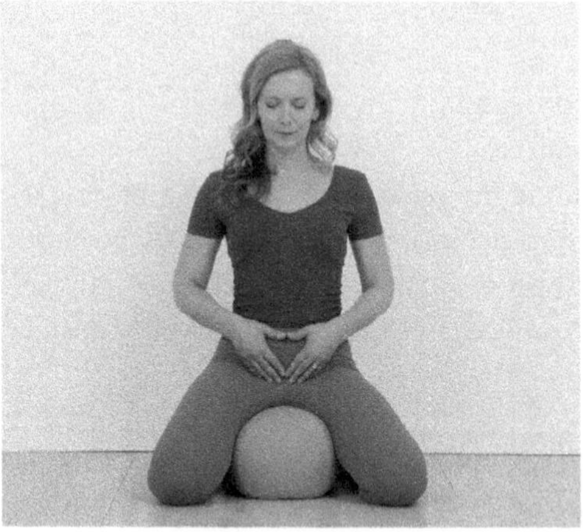

Hands in yoni mudrā on the lower abdomen

Let's start exploring from below. Think of the pelvic diaphragm (also referred to as the pelvic floor). Here you have the entrance to the vagina. Towards the top of the vaginal canal, you have the cervix, which is the lower part of the uterus. I interchange the words uterus and womb. They are the same. The uterus is sometimes said to be the shape and size of an upside-down pear – or maybe an avocado. This is where much of the action happens when it comes to the menstrual cycle. We will return here in a moment.

On either side of the uterus, you have the uterine tubes. You may know them as Fallopian tubes named after anatomist Gabriele Falloppio, but I like the anatomical descriptive name rather than the name of the male anatomist. The uterine tubes extend towards the two ovaries, one on the right, and one on the left. The ovaries are not attached to the uterine tubes but the fingerlike fimbria at the end of the uterine tubes catch the eggs from the ovaries every month. The ovaries are held in place by ligaments attached to the womb. This includes the broad ligament, the more specific ovarian ligament and the suspensory ligament. The ligaments also form attachments to the pelvic and abdominal walls.

The pelvic organs

The oval-shaped ovaries produce the hormones oestrogen and progesterone. They also mature an egg, oocyte (an immature egg cell), mid-cycle every month. This is ovulation.

Let's get back to the womb space, the uterus.

The uterus sits between the bladder and the rectum. It has several ligaments holding it in place. These include the broad ligament, round ligament and cardinal ligaments as well as the pubocervical and uterosacral ligaments. The top part of the uterus is called the fundus, then we have the body of the uterus, and the bottom part connecting it and opening up to the vagina is the cervix.

The inside of the uterus is covered by the endometrium or uterine lining. Every month it builds up during the follicular phase, or the first part of the cycle, and then it releases again as part of menstruation. Outside the endometrium, we have another layer called the myometrium. The outermost layer is the perimetrium.

The uterus is an incredible muscle. By weight, it is the strongest in the body, with its ability to contract and release in order to grow and birth a baby. The uterus supports a whole new organ – the placenta – when pregnant, and it grows and releases the uterine lining every month. The uterus is pretty special.

The uterus is also innervated (supplied with nerves) through the hypogastric nerve and pelvic splanchnic nerves, connecting to both the sympathetic and parasympathetic systems. It is connected to the central nervous system through the vagus nerve.

Understanding that our nervous system and the uterus are connected can inform how we teach our yoga classes or one-to-one sessions. If we regulate the nervous system and activate the vagus nerve how does this affect the uterus and therefore menstruation? I cannot find any specific research on this (yet). But we can speculate on how balancing our nervous system can have a potentially profound effect on our cycle, fertility and beyond. As we move into physiology, we will also notice that stress does, in fact, affect our hormones and therefore our cycle too.

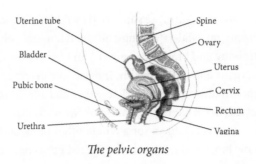

These organs and structures are supported by the pelvic floor, also known as the pelvic diaphragm. Understanding a bit about how our pelvic diaphragm moves with our body and breath also give us an idea of how important it is for our pelvic organs and pelvic health. Indeed, our pelvic and respiratory diaphragms work in unison. They work together and affect each other; we'll talk more about this in Chapter 13. In this book, we won't discuss much about the pelvic floor. That is a subject for a whole other book and something I write about in my blogs and discuss in my Sacred Pelvis online immersion.

Everything is connected, and healthy pelvic organs are supported by a healthy pelvic diaphragm, supported by the muscles, ligaments and fascia. If anything is too tight or doesn't give enough support to, say the uterus, it may affect the experience of the cycle, especially giving discomfort around the period.

If you love anatomy and physiology, you might also want to look further into the endopelvic fascia and how that connects to the rest of our body.

The *Āyurvedic* perspective on the anatomy of the female reproductive system is not dissimilar to the Western one described above. Any gynaecological reference is referred to as *strīroga* in *Āyurvedic* medicine. The word *yoni* refers to the female reproductive system: vulva, vagina, cervix, uterus, endometrium, ovaries and uterine tubes. This word is used in classical and newer *Āyurvedic* texts. In the *Caraka-saṃhitā*, there is a chapter devoted to *yonivyapat* or the 20 different disorders of the *yoni*. *Yoni* is another word adopted into the English language when talking about feminine energy and the female reproductive system.

You may have heard about *yoni mudrā* or various forms of *yoni mudrās* in yoga. This is sometimes referring specifically to how the *mudrā*, or hand gesture, symbolizes the *yoni*. Sometimes *yoni* is interpreted as the womb in female anatomy, which is the source of us as human beings growing in our mother's womb. It is also referred to as the womb or source of creation, the Cosmic womb. There are many variations of hand gestures or *mudrās* when it comes to *yoni mudrā* and we will explore these in a later chapter.

Energetic anatomy

As a yoga teacher, you may also be interested in the energetics of the pelvic area where we hold all our reproductive organs. Although not strictly yoga or *Āyurvedic* philosophy, the *cakras* or energetic wheels are popular with many yoga teachers and students.

We find references to these energetic centres in many contemporary books on yoga and they are most likely also mentioned in your yoga teacher training courses. Many references are a combination of Eastern philosophy and newer concepts of the energy body rather than traditional (mostly) *Tantrik* teachings. The *Tantrik* and classical scriptures may have a different take on the commonly known rainbow colours and physical areas of the *cakras*. The *cakras* and energetics are just that: energetic and spiritual connections, not a physical place in the body. Even so, the newer and less yogīc/*Tantrik* interpretations of the *cakras* are also valid and a great (and simpler) way to understand how yoga is not just a physical exercise or stretching technique but something that affects us emotionally, mentally and energetically. Yoga is a path on our spiritual evolutionary journey.

So what are the cakras?

We can say the *cakras* are energetic or spiritual centres associated with different areas of our physical body. Again, please note that many of the traditional yogīc and *Tantrik* texts will be very different from what we popularly discuss as the *cakra* system today.

There are many *cakras*, although most of us are only familiar with six or seven. These *cakras* are thought to be where main *nadis*, or energetic channels, meet. The main channel is *sushumna nadi*, associated with the spine, and *pingala* and *ida nadi*, which intertwine from one side to the other, much like a helix.

Starting at the base of the spine we have the main *cakras*:

- The root, *mūlādhāra* at the base of the spine, the perineum or the cervix in female anatomy, depending on the source.
- The sacral *cakra*, *svādhiṣṭhāna* behind the pubic bones towards the spine or sacrum.
- The navel centre, *maṇipūra cakra*.
- The heart area is called *anāhata*.
- The throat is *viśuddhi cakra*.
- The third eye centre is *ājñā cakra*.
- The *sahasrāra cakra* is the crown of the head but it's debatable if this is even an actual *cakra* or a different energetic connection.

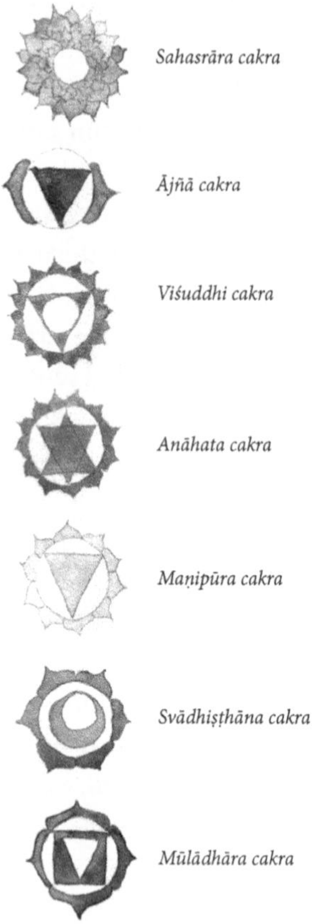

The common symbolism and interpretation of the cakra system

If we consider the so-called physical locations of the *mūlādhāra* and *svādhiṣṭhāna cakra* in the pelvic bowl they most certainly have an emotional-mental connection with the menstrual cycle and how we feel about our cyclic nature. Perhaps even to our gender and history, or rather herstory.

The elements of the cakras

Remember the five elements from the *Sāṅkhya* philosophy? Space, air, fire, water and earth. These five elements are related to the *cakras*: earth to the root *cakra*, water to the sacral *cakra*, fire to the navel area, air to the heart and space to the throat. Anything beyond that is beyond the elements and physical manifestations.

The root *cakra* associated with the element of earth is a place of stability, support and feeling safe. It is where we ground ourselves, the connection to our home, security, family or community.

Many of us feel ungrounded, we have lost connection to our land and ancestry, our history (or herstory) and with the wise elders of our culture. Even the connection to the menstrual cycle has been taken away through hormonal contraception and having to be more linear rather than cyclical.

I love that in the textbook physiological birth, the baby will come into this world with their crown (*cakra*) first through the birthing parent's root (*cakra*), connecting the two.

Perhaps these are some of the contemplations we can consider when we teach yoga for the cyclic nature.

The sacral *cakra* is interesting too when it comes to our cyclic nature. In some texts, it is said to be associated with the cervix. This is the bottom part of the uterus and the opening into the vagina.

The element is water and water is fluidity, juiciness and flow, and includes saliva. No saliva, no taste and therefore no pleasure. The energetics of the sacral *cakra* are connected to pleasure and taste – finding one's creative expression, sexuality, sensuality and a sense of one's own wants and needs.

We are often taught to feel shameful around the menstrual cycle and bleeding time. Shame about pleasure and sex. For many cultures, these topics still carry a huge stigma. But things are changing with people starting to be more vocal around menstruation, the cycles and feeling sensual and sexual.

If you like working with the *cakras* and incorporating them into your yoga practice or teachings you might want to reflect on some of these ideas when you share about working with our cyclical nature, our physiology and energy.

Even for the sceptics of energetic concepts, it is now accepted that emotions and our mental wellbeing are affected by our physiology, and similarly our mental health affects our physiology. This includes the hormones as well as the nervous system, and the vagus nerve which is connected to the uterus, as described earlier. We also understand that stress and anxiety affect our breathing. They affect our muscle tonicity, including that of the pelvic floor. And we know that our respiratory diaphragm and pelvic diaphragm are connected too. We have fascial and muscular links that enforce this physical connection.

Our yoga practice and teaching can affect all these different layers and aspects of our students through our intention, words, sequencing, choice of poses and the connection we have with the students or clients.

Everything is connected.

Female versus male alignment in yoga

At the beginning of the book, we discussed how today's yoga classes are inspired and influenced mostly by male teachers such as K. Pattabhi Jois, B.K.S. Iyengar and Swami Sivananda.

The story goes that many of the common alignment cues we use in our modern flow or *vinyāsa* classes came from K. Pattabhi Jois and the Mysore *Aṣṭāṅga Vinyāsa* yoga. Most of us have been in one such class or perhaps we teach these specific alignment cues. Common instructions include aligning the feet heel to heel, or heel to arch in *vīrabhadrāsana* (warrior poses).

It is said that this style of yoga was at one point taught mainly to Indian teenage boys in India during K. Pattabhi Jois's appointment at the Sanskrit College in Mysore, India. This is most likely true, although whether this influenced the *Aṣṭāṅga Vinyāsa* specific alignment I cannot say. Regardless, males, especially Indian teenage boys, have very different anatomy from the average female body with her wider pelvis.

I am sharing this story because it is worth asking why. Why do we tell our students certain alignment cues, why do their feet need to be facing a certain way, why do the feet and knees need to be together? Having taught many pregnancy and postnatal yoga teacher training courses for qualified yoga teachers, I have often had this discussion. In pregnancy and postnatal yoga we start to modify our alignment cues to support the changing and growing bodies of our pregnant students.

Coming back to the alignment cues that in *vīrabhadrāsana* (warrior poses), the heels need to be aligned with each other. Or perhaps the front heel should be aligned with the inner arch of the back foot. Is this specific alignment working for everybody? If you have a wider pelvis, sacroiliac joint issues or need to be mindful of your ankle and knee joints, does this alignment sound supportive to the body? Perhaps the feet need to be wider, perhaps the stance has to be shorter to stabilize the joints of the ankles, knees and sacroiliac joints. This is not just about the pregnant body. It is about how all bodies vary and certainly how male and female anatomical structures differ.

It's not only the wider pelvis of the female anatomy but also the effect it has on the rest of the body such as the knees in comparison with the male anatomy that should be considered. The so-called Q-angle, or quadriceps angle, is wider in the female body than the male. This angle is measured from lines drawn from the anterior superior iliac spine to the centre of the patella and from the centre of the patella to the tibial tuberosity. This angle is wider in female than male anatomy. It may affect knee health and knee alignment, as well as how the glutes, piriformis and quadriceps stretch and align.

And perhaps it may even affect the movement of the feet. Considering that most sports science research and papers use data on males, we are losing out on how people with female anatomy could be supporting, strengthening and understanding their anatomy and training better. Please see the section 'New research and lack of research' in Chapter 10 for further references on gender bias in sports and medical sciences.

If you consider this difference between male and female anatomy, how would you modify your yoga teaching? And what about your own yoga practice compared to what you may read in some resources and books or have heard from your teachers?

The breasts are another obvious anatomical difference and in the menstrual cycle they can change in sensitivity and size. This is another thing to consider when we teach the female body. The curvature of the spine, how we grow muscle tissue, even the capacity of the lungs, are different between the sexes. The female hormones affect the ligaments and physiology differently from the male hormones in the male body. There are many other differences but these are beyond the scope and subject of this book.

If you have been told to teach a certain way and that this is the only way to align and cue the yoga poses, it is challenging to change. This is especially true for newer teachers who have been taught a very specific sequence with specific alignment cues, or if you follow certain traditions of yoga.

As we start to teach differently shaped bodies, people who have less or more body awareness, strong and flexible bodies and tighter more constricted bodies of all ages and abilities, we learn how to adapt. We need to look at the individual person to modify and support that specific body. And, more importantly, we must invite our students to notice what is right for them.

This is the same when we start to explore how to work with our cyclic nature and *Āyurveda* in the yoga practice. I offer a template and inspiration from my own experience, as a yoga practitioner, a yoga teacher and from an *Āyurvedic* perspective, but everybody is different and we and our students must learn to accommodate own experience and body.

All I ask is for you to consider why a certain yoga pose, flow or alignment is the best option for a specific student – or yourself. Is there a way to adjust, modify and enhance the experience?

CHAPTER 7

Western Physiology and Hormones

The Western medical view of the cycle

Although we are looking through the *Āyurvedic* lens, when it comes to the cycle and yoga we also need to discuss the Western view of hormones and physiology.

This is the language most of us and our students are familiar with. It is the language your students will understand until you educate them from an *Āyurvedic* perspective. If they have a diagnosis, it will also be worded from a Western science view of hormones and physiology.

But do you remember anything from your biology lessons when it comes to the menstrual cycle? Were you even taught about the cycle in school or your yoga training? We will go through the very basics and then we will apply the Western language to the art and science of *Āyurveda* and yoga in the next chapter, and refer back to it as we discuss yoga, *Āyurveda* and the cycle.

What is the menstrual cycle?

The cycle starts on the first day of the bleed, or the period; this is counted as day 1. The cycle lasts until the day before you bleed again. To clarify, the menstrual cycle is the whole length of menstruation, follicular phase, ovulation and luteal phase. It is not just menstruation or the period. You may also hear it referred to as the ovulatory cycle or fertility cycle. The cycle refers to hormonal fluctuations and changes. Perhaps the main events are menstruation and ovulation. But there are shifts throughout the cycle.

As we mentioned in Chapter 5 on the moon cycle, the lunation, or lunar month, is 29.5 days. If the cycle is anywhere from approximately 25–30 days, it is considered normal. In a textbook, a cycle is referred to as 28 days but that only applies to about 13 per cent of menstruating people (Soumpasis, Grace

& Johnson 2020). It is also worth remembering that many don't a have 100 per cent regular cycle. It is sometimes a little longer or shorter than usual.

The menstrual cycle is a hormonal event, or rather a host of many hormonal events, and is divided into four main phases.

Phase 1: Menstruation (in some texts this is also the early follicular phase)

Phase 2: Follicular phase

Phase 3: Ovulation phase

Phase 4: Luteal phase

There are several hormones at play during the menstrual cycle. Let's look at some of the common ones.

Prostaglandins

These are hormone-like chemicals and part of the initiation of menstruation. Prostaglandins are generally released in any area of damage or infection in the body, including the cells and tissues in the uterus. Prostaglandins are part of the healing process and can cause inflammation and pain.

Oestrogen

This is often referred to as a female hormone. There are several oestrogens. Generally, these are the hormones that make us feel good by boosting the neurotransmitters serotonin and dopamine. These neurotransmitters make us feel happier and create a sense of wellbeing and pleasure. Oestrogen increases the uterine lining to prepare for ovulation and potential pregnancy. Other roles include muscle health, brain, sleep and heart health. Oestrogen also benefits bones, which is why the decrease in oestrogen during the perimenopause and menopause is a concern for osteoporosis.

Follicle-stimulating hormone

This pituitary hormone stimulates the ovarian follicles to mature. This in turn starts to release estradiol which is one of the oestrogens in the body.

Luteinising hormone

The luteinising hormone triggers ovulation as it releases an egg from its follicle. The egg is caught by the fimbriae of the uterine tubes. This egg is now ready for potential fertilization.

Corpus luteum

This is the endocrine gland formed by the empty egg follicle after ovulation. The corpus luteum starts to secrete the hormone progesterone.

Progesterone

This hormone is often likened to a chill-out and relaxing hormone. It counters some of the more energizing qualities of oestrogen. Where oestrogen builds up the endometrium, progesterone maintains it to prepare for a potentially fertilized egg to be implanted. Progesterone also reduces cervical mucus, whereas oestrogen increases it.

The hormones and the menstrual cycle

Menstruation phase

Menstruation happens as we shed the uterine lining that has been built up in the womb during the previous cycle. The hypothalamus, pituitary gland and ovaries work together to release hormones that bring about the bleed.

A very simplified explanation is that progesterone levels drop at this time causing a lack of blood circulation to the endometrium. This causes a release of prostaglandins; this in turn makes the uterus contract and the endometrial tissues, which lacked blood supply, will be shed. The capillaries break, causing the bleeding, which is then mixed with the endometrial tissues.

Prostaglandins can cause inflammation, which leads to pain. If they enter the bloodstream they can lead to headaches, nausea and diarrhoea, all common complaints during menstruation. This means we might be more receptive or sensitive to pain during our period. We might have more achy muscles after an intense yoga class or workout than at other times in the cycle. One of the triggers starting this process is the corpus luteum. This is the ovum follicle, or egg, which has not been fertilized. It is then reabsorbed into the body. Progesterone falls and then the spiral arteriole in the uterus starts to constrict as the build-up of lining is no longer needed.

As menstruation begins we are at the lowest levels of progesterone and oestrogen. We may feel fatigued, tired and nauseous and have period pain. The average length of this phase is four to six days with around 30ml of menstrual fluid being considered normal.

Menstruation is, in fact, the start of the follicular phase and the beginning of a new cycle.

Follicular phase

In medical language, the follicular phase starts on the first day of the period and lasts until ovulation. In this, and many other, books and literature, we honour the menstrual phase as a separate part of the cycle.

When the period ends, the endometrium is already in the process of renewing and rebuilding inside the uterus. The endometrium, or uterine lining, from a procreation perspective, supports and holds a fertilized egg and a potential pregnancy.

But it is so much more than that.

Towards the end of the bleed, the follicle-stimulating hormone starts to increase. It facilitates the maturation of the ovum or egg. It is one of these eggs that will eventually ovulate at the ovulatory phase. However, it takes around 100 days for the follicle to mature so any issues around this phase may only manifest a few months later.

This process releases the hormone oestrogen, mainly a type of oestrogen called estradiol. This in turn starts the process of increasing the endometrial lining in the womb. This is the lining that will be shed during the following menstruation. The increasing oestrogen will give us more energy after our period. We feel stronger and more motivated with the increased oestrogen levels. Oestrogen is important for our bone health, brain and heart and it influences sleep too.

Although sports research on this specific topic is scant and can be contradictory there are some suggestions that this is a time where we can favour building up muscle and strength (Romero-Moraleda *et al.* 2019).

Ovulation

Just before we ovulate, the luteinising hormone (LH) increases sharply and an egg is released for potential fertilization. This happens around mid-cycle or in a textbook cycle on day 14. But, one may have a shorter or longer follicular cycle and therefore a different day of ovulation. It can happen from either the right or left ovary, in no specific pattern.

Oestrogen also increases just before and around ovulation. Remember that oestrogen is the feminine hormone giving us glow, confidence and sensuality? Well, research shows that lap dancers get more tips during ovulation than at any other time in their cycle (Miller, Tybur & Jordan 2007). Perhaps this is confirmation that the female body shows it is fertile at the time. It might also be that the hormones give us more confidence or openness to please others and ourselves. Maybe we feel more attractive or are more attracted to others, just as it seems others are attracted to us (or those visiting lap dancing clubs are attracted to the ovulating dancer).

There are some suggestions (Wojtys *et al.* 1998) that anterior crucial ligament (knee) injury is higher at this time in female athletes, potentially because of laxity in the joints due to hormonal changes. Again, the evidence is inconclusive.

Ovulation is literally a one-day event. The egg releases and this is the only time in the phase you can get pregnant. However, sperm can live inside the female reproductive system for around five days. So those days up to and including ovulation make up the so-called fertile window.

The feeling of sensuality, confidence and energy when our oestrogen levels are high is also what we will refer to as the ovulation phase as we move through this book.

Luteal phase

After the release of the egg during ovulation, the follicle transforms into the corpus luteum, an endocrine gland, which will start to produce the hormone progesterone. This process peaks in the mid-luteal phase. As progesterone is at a higher level than oestrogen, we have less capacity to please others and don't have the same energy and motivation. We can say the rose-tinted glasses of oestrogen have been taken off and we see things a little more clearly.

If pregnancy occurs, progesterone will be there to support the fertilized egg in the early stages of pregnancy. As our cycle continues and no pregnancy occurs, progesterone drops again and the period will soon start. Progesterone slows and calms things down. We might have constipation as the peristalsis of our intestines can slow down.

We may find our coordination is more challenging and there could be longer reaction time in this phase when it comes to sports and exercise. Our temperature also rises during the luteal phase. This can disturb our sleep and certainly if you do any intense workouts you need to be mindful of staying hydrated and cooling down again. As you move closer to your period you may start to feel fatigued and tired due to the drop in hormones.

And so the cycle starts again

We are all individuals and unique and these are just some of the hormonal shifts occurring during our monthly cycle. As we look into the *Āyurvedic* physiology you will see how similar it is. But, as always, we all experience our hormones and cycles differently. There is no way it should be or should feel. The main thing is that you, and your students, observe their shifts and then work with their cycle rather than against it or simply ignore these changes. This is what you are learning as you read this book.

CHAPTER 8

Āyurvedic Physiology and the Menstrual Phases

How *Āyurveda* views the menstrual cycle

Āyurvedic physiology isn't that different from what is described in the Western chapter on the menstrual cycle phases. *Āyurveda* may use different terminology or words but in essence, it is very similar.

As students of yoga, we can also say that Western science works on the level of the gross physical body or the *sthulaśarīra*, whereas *Āyurveda* additionally includes the subtle body or *sūkṣmaśarīra*. The subtle body is where we find the *manas* (mind), *buddhi* (intellect) and the five elements which we discovered in the *Sāṅkhya* philosophy section.

You may want to earmark the introduction to *Āyurveda* in Chapter 3 as we will refer back to the *doṣas*, the qualities of the *doṣas* and the movement of *vāyu* or *prāṇa* in this chapter. We will also discover some new words from *Āyurvedic* terminology.

In *Āyurveda*, we say the body is made out of seven tissues or structures called *dhātus*. We have *rasa* (plasma), *rakta* (blood), *māṃsa* (muscle), *meda* (adipose tissue), *asthi* (bones), *majjā* (bone marrow) and *śukra* in male physiology and *ārtava* in female physiology. *Śukra* and *ārtava* are our reproductive tissues respectively. We will discuss *ārtava dhātu* in terms of our menstrual cycle.

Āyurveda is a holistic system and for healthy *dhātus* we need to start with how we nourish ourselves. The food we consume needs to be well digested and then the qualities and nourishment from what we consume moves through the tissues, or *dhātus*, in the order described in the previous paragraph. This process takes about 35 days. What nourished (or depleted) your *rasa dhātu* takes 35 days to get to your *ārtava dhātu* (Lad 2002). What we did a month ago will show up in our cycle and reproductive health but not necessarily immediately. Remember from our Western physiology that it takes about

100 days for the follicle to mature, so any issues around this time may only manifest a few months later. This is good to remember and to let our students know. Although we might feel an immediate effect on some levels when we practise yoga, it is a long-term practice. It can take time to see the effect in our cycle.

The *dhātus* also become affected by the *doṣas*. If a *doṣa* moves into a *dhātu* it may present symptoms or become a dis-ease. For example, *kapha doṣa* is heavy, sluggish and symbolizes build-up. If *kapha* comes into *ārtava dhātu* there might be an obstruction to the regular movement and flow of *vāta* or *prāṇa*, perhaps leading to excess growth such as polycystic ovary syndrome.

Ārtavacakra – the menstrual cycle and seasons

In *Āyurveda* we call the menstrual cycle *ārtavacakra. Cakra* means a wheel and here it acknowledges the cyclic seasons of the monthly cycle or infradian rhythm. *Ārtava* is the female reproductive tissue. The word *ārtava* comes from the root *rtu* meaning season. As a side note, we have a concept called *ṛtucharyā* meaning a seasonal routine within the cycles of the year. In *Āyurveda*, we acknowledge that we need to adjust our habits, routines, what we eat and how we exercise according to the seasons. We can take this principle into the seasons of the menstrual cycle.

Just like the Western medical perspective *Āyurveda* also divides the cycle into different phases.

> *Rajahsrāvakāla* is menstruation.
>
> *Ṛtukāla* is the days after the bleed until ovulation – the follicular phase.
>
> *Beejotsarga* is ovulation and usually included in *ṛtukāla*.
>
> *Ṛtuvyatitakāla* is the luteal phase of the menstrual cycle.

Let's look at each phase in greater detail. You will get an understanding of the *Āyurvedic* and *doṣic* principles. This is the foundation for why we adjust our yoga practice according to *Āyurveda* through our menstrual cycle.

Menstruation or *rajahsrāvakāla*

Āyurveda has very specific descriptions of the perfect period. In the *Āyurvedic* classics, it says the colour of the blood should be bright red like that of rabbit blood or a red lotus flower. It shouldn't stain clothes or have a foul smell (although it will have an aroma). It should be clot-free. The amount according to the *Āyurvedic* classics is four *añjali*. One *añjali* is the amount you can have in your cupped hands. An ideal period would last three to five days. These specifications are referenced in both *Caraka-saṃhitā Cikitsasthana* and the *Aṣṭāṅga-hṛdayam Sarirasthana*.

You may remember that *vāta doṣa* has five *subdoṣas* or subtypes. The one we are mostly concerned with is *apāna vāyu*, the downward and outward moving aspect of the wind element and *vāta*. *Apāna vāyu* is responsible for the elimination of urine, faeces and menstrual fluid as well as childbirth and ejaculation, and is associated with our out-breath.

For healthy menstruation, we need *apāna vāyu* to be balanced. If there are any obstructions or imbalances here it will affect our flow. When we start to look at yoga poses and sequences we will learn what poses may support the flow of *apāna vāyu* and what may restrict it.

Because of this connection to *apāna vāyu* we say that *vāta doṣa* governs the menstruation phase of our cycle. *Vāta* is mobility. It makes things move. We need the function of *vāta* to move the menstrual fluid out of the uterus.

The *Āyurvedic* classics also discuss the menstrual cycle and menstruation in connection to conception. Given the time the classics were written down this makes sense. During this time, procreation and having a large family was important for one's social and financial support system, just like it was in many places in the world. However, we will not focus on the aim to become pregnant or pregnancy itself in this book. Rather, we'll acknowledge that the menstrual cycle is a vital sign of health and wellbeing. Remember that menstrual cycle health is important whether someone wants children or not.

Is menstruation dirty or a detox?

Menstruation isn't dirty but rather a very powerful function of the body. It is not toxic and we do not need to clean the womb from toxins. Even in *Āyurveda*, it's believed that when the *doṣas* and the digestive fire, *agni*, work well, the body will always want to find equilibrium. In Chapter 4 on the *Āyurvedic* view on menstruation, I mentioned the term *āma*, often translated as toxins. Perhaps a more correct interpretation is that *āma* is undigested material that can become sludge or toxic to the body. Menstruation isn't *āma*. But the menstrual blood and blood itself can carry *āma*.

In *Āyurveda*, there is a special cleansing regime called *pañchakarma*, which is a deep and long process of detox and healing. In some practices this includes bloodletting, called *raktamokṣa*. Bloodletting is prescribed by

Āyurvedic doctors for several complaints and conditions. It is a practice that is still used in *Āyurvedic* hospitals and by *Āyurvedic* doctors. Many cultures and traditions have used this treatment.

The blood tissue, or *rakta dhātu*, is the *dhātu* formed in the body after *rasa* or plasma. Where plasma and blood are often thought of together in Western physiology, they are separate but closely related in *Āyurveda*. They carry some hormones around the body and regulate our temperature. *Rakta dhātu* is our red blood cells and blood vessels. It is connected with *pitta doṣa* and the element of fire. Like all other *dhātus*, it can become vitiated and imbalanced. Things that may cause issues in *rakta dhātu* include hot and spicy food, alcohol, too much sun and heat. Emotions such as anger, envy and hate can also affect *rakta dhātu*. It's all about balance, though, because we want the healthy warm glow of *rakta* too.

Although any *doṣa* can affect the *dhātus*, it is often excess *pitta doṣa* that's found in the *rakta dhātu*. *Pitta* qualities include being ambitious, sharp and quick. It is the type-A personality much revered in our culture. *Pitta* people can do it all until they literally burn out. If you are a *pitta* constitution, if you live a *pitta* lifestyle or eat *pitta*-increasing food, this may affect your menstruation due to *pitta*'s relation to *rakta dhātu* and *rakta*'s association of being released through the menstrual blood.

If *rakta dhātu* is afflicted, one of the treatments could be *raktamokṣa*. In a way, this is what the menstrual cycle does. The body has an intelligent system of bloodletting every month. We don't need leeches (yes, leeches *are* still used for this treatment) or syringes to carry out the bloodletting – the menstrual cycle releases excess *pitta* or heat.

From this point of view, the bleed is a vital sign. If the body is functioning well it will try to create balance, and that may be through the period – a natural *raktamokṣa*.

Our periods give us incredible insight into our overall health and wellbeing. Everything is connected. What we eat, drink, smoke and feel will be expressed in our body and the period is one of the ways our body's intelligence speaks to us.

How the doṣas affect the menstrual phase

Because we are all unique beings with our own variations of the *doṣas* and susceptibility to *doṣic* imbalances, our periods will also have variants between us. We will look at a typical period according to the three *doṣas* and how they affect menstruation. Remember, these are generalizations and will differ from person to person. Whatever *doṣa* is prominent in you or your client, the bleeding time is always influenced by *apāna vāyu* and *vāta doṣa*.

Periods influenced by *vāta doṣa*

Vāta is light and irregular and that's how menstruation will present itself. The cycle may be shorter than 29 days or very irregular in length. The bleed is most likely short and light. Excess *vāta* is often associated with pain. Pain in the lower back and legs can be a symptom of excess *vāta doṣa*. *Vāta* may also manifest as insomnia and anxiety.

***Pitta*-affected periods**

Pitta is heat and fire. This can cause the bleed to be heavy and have a stronger scent. When we are too hot and have excess *pitta*, we may also feel irritation and anger, including premenstrual tension. Excess *pitta* could manifest as acne and diarrhoea. *Pitta doṣa* is sharp and quick so the menstrual cycle may be shorter than the textbook 28 days.

***Kapha*-dominant menstruation**

Kapha tends to accumulate. It is slow and dense. Periods influenced by *kapha* may manifest as heavy, mucousy, with a longer bleeding time. *Kapha* is very regular and steady so the cycle will be regular too.

Due to the *kapha* quality of accumulation, water retention can manifest in *kapha*-dominant people. A dull ache and a sense of heaviness are also *kapha* qualities. Tender and swollen breasts can be a symptom of *kapha*. Mentally this can manifest as feeling low or depressed.

The follicular phase or *rutakala*

This phase starts from the end of menses and includes ovulation. It is the fertile window where there is potential for pregnancy. As in the Western perspective, this is the time when we build up the uterine lining. But in *Āyurveda* we connect this time to *kapha doṣa*. *Kapha* is about building up, nourishment, support and stability. *Kapha* is therefore the *doṣa* responsible for preparing the uterus for potential conception. In a way, *kapha* is very similar to oestrogen.

Kapha supports the growth of muscles; it makes recovery easier and *kapha* has strength, steadiness and endurance. This is a perfect time to embrace those qualities. As we looked at hormones from a Western perspective, this is the phase where we might enjoy more physically demanding activities or more dynamic yoga practices with challenging strength-building *āsana*. One of *kapha*'s qualities is coolness and we can build up heat and sweat to balance the cool qualities of *kapha doṣa*.

Kapha sometimes has a bad reputation of being lazy, heavy and depressed. Although this may be true when it's imbalanced, the balanced *kapha* is love, compassion and beauty. This can be the grounded sensuality we need in the fertile window to either mate and procreate, to birth a project or new idea or simply to be in touch with our body and sense of pleasure. Because our culture appreciates the focused, ambitious and sharp qualities of *pitta* and the quick creative mind of *vāta*, we sometimes forget about the sustaining qualities of *kapha*. These are qualities of being embodied, nourishing our bodies and being present.

Ṛtuvyatitakāla – the luteal phase

Towards the end of *ṛtukāla*, or the follicular phase, *pitta doṣa* slowly starts to increase. My interpretation is that *pitta* gives the spark to start ovulation. *Pitta* is about transformation. The time between ovulation and menstruation is mostly influenced by *pitta*.

Where *kapha* helped to build up the endometrium, *pitta* helps to enhance the blood circulation in the uterine lining. This is to create a nurturing environment and the best possible space for a potential fertilized egg to grow and become a baby – if you try to conceive. This is the time progesterone starts to increase and we can perhaps see a correlation between *pitta* and progesterone here.

One of the positive qualities of *pitta* is the sharp clear focus, so this can be a great phase to focus on technique and alignment in the yoga *āsana* class.

As *pitta* is heat and fire it corresponds with the slight increase of our basal temperature. It is not the time to do hot yoga. Rather, make sure you are hydrated and enjoy a steady or even relaxed pace.

Excess *pitta* may manifest as inflammation, excess heat or hot flushes. Many of our common premenstrual complaints of irritation, anger and frustration are also related to increased *pitta*.

Remember, *pitta* is a natural influence at this time of the cycle but symptoms of excess *pitta* come from your lifestyle, routine, the food you eat, the beverages you drink, including alcohol, and whether you embrace a *pitta* or type-A personality. This also reflects the *pitta* mind of anger and irritation. Yoga can be one of the tools to calm any heated emotions and excess *pitta* qualities in the mind.

We all have a unique cycle

It is worth remembering that there are so many things happening all the time in our physiology and energy. All the *doṣas* play a role throughout the cycle. I have chosen to focus on just a few *Āyurvedic* aspects for each of the phases as a guide to how to approach our yoga *āsana* practice.

The menstrual cycle manifests differently from person to person and month to month. We are all unique and we all have our own physiological, mental, emotional, cultural and spiritual associations and experiences when it comes to the cycle. It is our individual experience. But according to *Āyurveda*, if we are completely balanced, well and healthy, our periods and cycle should be pain free, regular and easy.

Now we know what *doṣas* and therefore what elements govern each phase of the cycle, we can consider how we want to enhance our yoga practice, working with our body rather than against its natural rhythms.

Keep all of this in mind when we move to the chapters on teaching yoga according to the menstrual cycle.

We also appreciate that we and our yoga students highly likely have some imbalances in the *doṣas* that will influence the cycle. We may not be in a position to diagnose these (unless you are an *Āyurvedic* practitioner qualified to do so) but we can utilize our experience, research and knowledge as we start to teach *Āyurvedic* cycle aware yoga. If we teach one-to-one sessions, we can get feedback and follow our observations closely during our yoga sessions with our clients.

The lunar cycle everyone can follow

We discussed the actual moon or lunar cycle and how it relates to the menstrual cycle in Chapter 5. Here is a reminder of the energetic potential for the different moon and menstrual cycle phases. Perhaps this can be an inspiration, whether you teach a menstrual cycle aware class, incorporate the lunar phases in your classes or teach yoga students who do not have a menstrual cycle.

New/dark moon

The sky is still dark. There is a sense of retreat and introspection in the darkness. Yet a new moon cycle is about to begin. So although we are in the darkness and in a place of rejuvenation and rest it is also a time to reflect on what we are opening up to for this new lunar month. Just like menstruation, it is time to dive deep, look inside and contemplate in a place of rest and retreat.

Waxing moon

The reflection of the moon starts to increase, just like the endometrium starts to build up after the menstrual phase. In *Āyurveda*, it is the *kapha* time of growth, stability and endurance. From a lunar perspective, this is where we can plant seeds of intention. As we plant the seeds they will grow just as the moon is growing in the sky. Anything we are looking to manifest and build up in abundance has the waxing moon energy to support it.

This is the fertile window of manifestation. In the menstrual cycle, this could mean building up an environment where sperm can stay alive and well until ovulation and potential conception. Energetically it could be the potential for any kind of creation or manifestation in our life. A new project, a painting, poem, an intention to grow financially or in health or be able to share our offerings abundantly.

Full moon

The glowing, illuminating and abundant full moon is ripe and fertile, just like ovulation. There might be a lot of superstition around the full moon and, for me, it does feel magical and very special. It is only 100 per cent full for a short moment, just as the actual ovulation only happens for about a day.

This is the time of manifestation in lunar magic. If a baby was to manifest in the womb this would be the time it would happen. Again we, or our students, may not want to become pregnant but it has that potential. Energetically, we all have the potential to manifest at this time or, as my yoga teacher Shiva Rea would say, 'We are all pregnant with potential'. The energy is high.

Waning moon

The moon slowly starts to get smaller again. It is waning. In the menstrual cycle, this is the luteal phase where we start to release and let go, where the body surrenders to either preparing for a new cycle or being pregnant. Energetically, this is also a letting-go phase. The sky is darker as the moon gets smaller in appearance. We can release what we no longer need, we can sort out, organize and let go.

As we move closer to the darkest part of the moon phases we feel the need to retreat and go within again, just as we might do as we approach the menstrual phase.

And so the outer and inner lunar cycle continues.

Following our personal pattern

I am aware that most of those who menstruate rarely follow this specific pattern. We don't all start menstruating on the new moon and ovulate on the full moon. Most of us move between these pinnacles of the moon phases because our cycle is rarely 29.5 days like the moon. Some seem to ovulate closer to the new moon and menstruate around the full moon. And most of us have cycles that move between them.

Perhaps when we had no light pollution, when we lived more in sync with the seasons and cycles of nature, we had this pattern. Perhaps when the time of introspection at the darkness of the new moon was honoured we too had space to surrender, rest and release our blood.

As yoga teachers and yoga practitioners, we can always connect with the actual moon cycles if we feel drawn to do so. If we or our students do not have a menstrual cycle this is a beautiful and nurturing practice to follow. Connecting with the actual moon and her changing phases.

CHAPTER 9

From Menarche to Menopause

The menstruating years

The menstrual cycle generally starts between the ages of 10 and 16, but most commonly at around 12 years old. The first period is called menarche, or *rajodarśana* in *Āyurvedic* medicine.

You already know the complexity of the hormones involved in the menstrual cycle. But factors such as having enough nutrition and weight are also part of the puzzle of when we start our cycle.

The classic *Āyurvedic* text the *Aṣṭāṅga-hṛdayam Sarīrasthāna* explains that '*rajas* (menstruation) which is the product of *rasa* (the first *dhātu*) flows out of the body for three days, every month, after the age of twelve years old and undergoes diminision [sic] by the age of fifty years'. The *Suśrutasaṃhitā śarīrasthāna* explains how the 'process (menstruation) commences at the twelfth year, flowing once a month, and continues till the fiftieth year'. It will manifest differently depending on one's unique constitution and dominant *doṣas*.

The Āyurvedic menarche

Vāta constitutions or imbalanced *vāta* are often more erratic, anxious and worried than other *doṣas*. Sometimes they are so busy in their own minds that they forget to eat and they lose weight easily. In case they have low body weight they may start their cycles on the latter end of the average. However, because of *vāta*'s irregularity, they may also start early.

The fiery *pitta doṣa* is quick and sharp, leading to earlier menarche. *Pitta* also has an association with *rakta dhātu*, the blood tissue, and hormones in general. The urban environment, with its busyness, full diary of activities and ambition, is also increasing *pitta* in our children, which may be a reason as to why menarche seems to start earlier than in previous generations. Having said that, healthy *pitta* people are well-balanced, healthy individuals and their fertile cycle could be very average and balanced too.

Slow and steady *kapha doṣa* people will patiently wait for their cycles to begin. *Kapha* is slow and can stagnate, which is why their menarche may be in the latter range. So although *kapha* people may appear strong and with a healthy weight, it is not all about adequate body weight.

Menarche as a rite of passage

Menarche is a very important time. A time of transition, of coming of age. Many cultures and traditions have some sort of celebration or ritual as children enter adulthood.

In my own culture, there isn't any acknowledgement of menarche. It may have been absorbed by the Christian rite of confirmation in the protestant church. However, there wasn't any celebration or congratulations when it came to my first period. To be honest, I would probably have been too embarrassed, but perhaps that is also an issue. Menstruation was neither anything dirty nor taboo when I grew up – it wasn't something we did not talk about. But it was also not something we *did* talk about.

When I was an apprentice in India for my postgraduate *Āyurveda* degree I became friends with some local young women. When one of them shared her photo albums she showed me pictures of a big celebration party. Everybody was dressed up, delicious food was served and my new friend looked like the star of the show. And she was. This was the celebration of her starting her menstrual cycle.

I do believe all cultures must have honoured this time as a rite of passage at some point in their history. Some still do. Many don't.

I love the acknowledgement and honouring of such a powerful time in a young person's life. In her book *Women's Power to Heal Through Inner Medicine*, Maya Tiwari (Mayatitananda 2007) also shares *Vedic* rituals to celebrate menarche. In modern-day Britain, women, such as Alexandra Pope and Sjanie Hugo Wurlitzer of Red School (Pope & Wurlizter 2017), share the importance of how our experience of our first bleed may influence how we view and experience our menstrual cycle for the rest of our life. We can now find people facilitating menarche rituals either retrospectively or for those 'coming of age'.

How does this affect your yoga teaching or indeed your yoga practice?

Modern yoga (physical *āsana* classes) has been shown again and again to improve our physical and emotional wellbeing. As you will see later, research shows that yoga can reduce menstrual cramps, pain as well as PMS and potentially be an alternative to painkillers.

If we introduce yoga to older children and adolescents before they start their cycle they will already have powerful tools and techniques to support them at this time of transition and change. Being a teenager, one has to adjust physically and mentally to the physiological and hormonal changes. Using yoga as a way to navigate through this time emotionally as well as physically can be a powerful support.

Yoga is also an excellent way to notice the changes in our physical body as well as emotionally without judgement. It can become a meditative mindful practice. When we start to bleed, we can use the practice of menstrual cycle awareness and practising with our cyclic nature to potentially reduce any symptoms of pain or discomfort.

I am not a specialist in yoga for children or teenagers so if you choose to work with adolescents you may need further training and research.

It can take a few years for our hormones to find their particular rhythm. The *doṣas* also shift from the childhood qualities of *kapha doṣa*, building up and growing to the adulthood of fire and ambition of *pitta*. All changes, especially sudden changes, are initiated by *vāta doṣa*. Consider the external environment. Are you in a stressful, busy, loud and noisy urban environment which may increase *vāta* and/or *pitta doṣa*? Or are you in a cool, damp place in the countryside where it's quiet and slow, which has more *kapha* qualities?

The menstruating years when there is no cycle

A regular cycle will become the norm for the next 40 years or so. If you become pregnant, give birth, take hormones such as the contraceptive pill, have an implant or some other medications and surgical procedures you may experience pauses from the menstrual cycle.

Periods and the fertile cycle may also stop if your body weight is too low to sustain a cycle, as can happen with anorexia. In sport, you may see people training and using more energy than they take in. This is referred to as relative energy deficiency in sports (RED-S) which can also cause the cycle to stop.

Transition to the wise woman years

The menopause is a very short event. It is the day when we haven't had a period for one whole year. The average age for this is at 51 years in the UK. After that day, we are postmenopausal. The time leading up to and around the menopause is called the perimenopause (National Health Service 2018).

The menopause can also happen earlier for various reasons. This could be due to certain cancer treatments. Radiotherapy may affect the cycle, and some chemotherapy can affect the ovaries and the cycle will stop. Surgery and removal of the uterus or ovaries in a hysterectomy will also trigger the menopause. Certain chromosome abnormalities and autoimmune diseases can stop ovarian functions and induce the menopause early.

Menopausal symptoms

Menopausal symptoms are generally perimenopausal symptoms. Peri means around. So perimenopause is the time around the menopause, although we generally use the term perimenopause for the time before our periods cease. This transition usually takes around five years but could be longer or shorter. We may also experience various symptoms post-menopause.

Hot flushes, night sweats, irritability, mood swings, depression, brain fog, vaginal dryness and low libido are all associated with the perimenopause. In many ways, your premenstrual symptoms are often showing up here.

During the perimenopause, the length of the cycles may become longer or shorter. You may not bleed for several months and suddenly have a cycle again. You may or may not ovulate as regularly as the hormones shift. Some people report that their periods are lighter and shorter. And for some, they become heavier and longer. All these changes and irregularities are associated with *vāta*. *Vāta* is the *doṣa* of change and instability.

From an *Āyurvedic* view, every sudden change is initiated by *vāta doṣa*. Moving from midlife to the next stage of life is a move from the *pitta*-influenced, ambitious, focused and outgoing lifestyle to a more contemplative, spiritual-seeking *vāta*-influenced phase. As we grow older, *vāta doṣa* will naturally influence our life.

Vāta is light, dry and rough. Excess *vāta* can cause our bones to become brittle leading to osteopenia and osteoporosis. This is another potential change as we grow older.

You may notice that many of the perimenopausal symptoms are associated with the hot and sharp *pitta*: hot flushes, irritability and night sweats. Heat can dry out the natural lubrication of the vagina. These are *pitta* symptoms which we, as yoga teachers, can cool down with *pitta*-reducing yoga, breathing or lifestyle changes. This would include lunar, *yin*-style yoga, restorative and calming practices, cooling breathing practices and mindfulness.

You may wonder why perimenopause symptoms are associated with *pitta* since we are transitioning into a *vāta* stage of life. I believe it's because our lifestyle generates a lot of *pitta*. We work hard and play hard. We are busy and stressed, always *doing* something. Our lifestyle increases *pitta doṣa*, as does our food: red meat, alcohol, coffee and cheese are all *pitta* increasing.

This build-up of *pitta* has to manifest somehow. It could be during the premenstrual phase or as perimenopause complaints. We are focusing on reproductive health but the *doṣas* can manifest in other ways as well, not just around the menstrual cycle.

Managing the *doṣas* and perimenopause

From an *Āyurvedic* perspective, *vāta* is always the initiator and needs to be addressed through *vāta*-reducing yoga practices and lifestyle changes. Then treat the *pitta*-related symptoms with cooling practices or, if you feel more *kapha* dominant, make sure *kapha* is reduced in lifestyle and diet.

To pacify excess *vāta* in our yoga practice, we can encourage a slow, steady breath. This encourages calming the mind to calm the body. Practising mindfulness has been seen to alleviate several perimenopausal symptoms such as hot flushes, depression and stress (Wong *et al.* 2018; van Driel *et al.* 2019).

Vāta-reducing yoga *āsana* are also slow and steady, calming the mind and body. It can be meditative and grounding. Yet, *vāta* also needs strength and stability. We need to build up juiciness, stamina, muscles and power, without exhausting ourselves. We also want to increase our *ojas*, rejuvenating immunity, which we discuss in Chapter 13 on the importance of rest.

Actual yoga *āsana* practice could reduce perimenopausal symptoms, stress levels and depression as well as increase quality of life. *Āsana* may also improve our balance and ability to move up and down from the ground, which is important as we get older and helps to prevent osteoporotic fractures (Jorge *et al.* 2016; Elavsky & McAuley 2007).

It is, as always, all about balance for the individual.

PART 3

TEACHING CYCLE-AWARE YOGA

CHAPTER 10

Bringing it All Together: Yoga, *Āyurveda*, Hormones and the Menstrual Cycle

I hope you now have more insight into how some of the hormonal and *doṣic* changes affect us and the menstrual cycle. If *Āyurveda* is new to you I trust you feel you have a good awareness of the basic principles of the sister science of yoga. It is my hope that you can implement this knowledge and how it affects the menstrual cycle into your yoga teaching and your personal practice if appropriate.

Remember that what we commonly refer to as the menstrual cycle is the whole cycle, rather than just the period itself.

We have discussed how both yoga and *Āyurveda* share the same principles and the same philosophy (*Sāṅkhya*). Now we want to look at how we can bring it all together.

Myth or fact?

Before we dive into how to teach cycle-aware yoga from an *Āyurvedic* perspective, I want to discuss some of the statements I have heard from yoga teachers, in yoga teacher trainings or in general yoga conversations about the menstrual cycle and yoga.

- Don't do inversions when you are on your period.

This is a common instruction given in yoga classes. However, if you ask the teacher, they often don't know why. It's just what they have been told, so they tell their students the same. It is always important to ask why, and why not.

And even when we ask and get an answer, it is worth using our discrimination and doing some research to see if the reasoning makes sense or not.

In this example, I have heard that inversions can make the blood flow back and can cause endometriosis or that the blood can clog up, and simply that it's bad for you. No reason was given.

From a Western medical perspective, there is absolutely no reason you shouldn't do inversions when menstruating. There is no more backflow than when lounging on the sofa. It won't cause endometriosis or any other gynaecological issues.

I have also heard that inversions can potentially damage the uterine ligaments, because the uterus may become larger and heavier during the period. There are two schools of thought on whether the uterus actually grows and becomes heavier during menstruation. Some say there is no evidence. Others say they are confident they can palpate how it changes during the cycle. Either way, it shouldn't have any negative effect on the uterine ligaments if you or your students were to invert during menstruation. The uterine ligaments have better elasticity than other ligaments and can extend and stretch perfectly. Just think of how much they need to stretch during pregnancy.

But let's look at it from an *Āyurvedic* perspective, in line with yoga philosophy and lifestyle.

Remember that menstruation is governed by *apāna vāyu*. *Apāna* is the downward flow of *prāṇa*, situated in the pelvis. From an *Āyurvedic* perspective, it is essential for our wellbeing that *apāna vāyu* is balanced. This will be reflected in how we experience menstruation.

If we move into an inversion such as *śīrṣāsana* (headstand), *sālamba-sarvāṅgāsana* (shoulderstand), *piñchamayūrāsana* (forearm stand) or *adhomukhavṛkṣāsana* (handstand) we are manipulating *apāna vāyu*. So, although our actual menstrual blood may not backflow, the energy of *apāna vāyu* may change direction. If this happens it can cause various health issues according to *Āyurveda*, which we will explore later.

If we apply *mūlabandha*, the root lock similar to a pelvic floor engagement, we are also manipulating the natural flow of *apāna vāyu* during menses. Often when we are in inversions we need that rooted stability to support the yoga pose, and *mūlabandha* is encouraged. This may be a good thing at other times. In yoga, we do connect with *mūlabandha* specifically to direct the energy upwards as a spiritual energetic practice. However, from a yoga and *Āyurvedic* view, this is not appropriate during our menstruation.

I consider poses such as *śīrṣāsana* (headstand), *sālambasarvāṅgāsana* (shoulderstand), *piñchhamayūrāsana* (forearmstand) and *adhomukhavṛkṣāsana* (handstand) as inversions, postures where you need engagement and direct the energy upwards. Looking at the subtle body, or the energetics, poses such as *adhomukhaśvānāsana* (downward-facing dog) aren't an inversion. Although we lift the pelvis we are grounding through the feet. It is the same in *viparīta karaṇī* (legs-up-the-wall), where we are releasing into the pelvis rather than bringing the engagement or energy up.

This is the reason yoga generally doesn't recommend inversions when you are on your period. I don't recommend anyone to be the 'yoga police'. We and our students know our own bodies the best and can take responsibility for our own bodies. In gymnastics, you won't hear a coach telling a gymnast off for doing flips, cartwheels and handstand contortions during their period. But from an energetic, yoga and *Āyurvedic* perspective, it is not advised.

- Don't engage the *bandhas*.

There are several *bandhas*, locks or seals, but I will focus on the *mūlabandha*. I mentioned *mūlabandha* in the discussion about inversions. *Mūla* means root and *bandha* is often translated as a seal or lock. *Mūlabandha* is sealing the root. For female anatomy, it is said that the *mūlabandha* is at the cervix, although some say the general area of the perineum or perineal body. For spiritual practices like meditations or *prāṇayāma*, we may connect to this area on an energetic rather than a physical level. It is a way for us to contain the energy generated from our practice rather than letting it flow out.

In *āsana* we can connect with the *bandha* as a pelvic floor engagement to support our physical posture.

Either way, during our period, the effect is that we lift and restrict the natural flow of *apāna vāyu* in its manifestation of menstruation. We naturally engage the pelvic floor spontaneously in certain movements and at specific times, like when we sneeze or lift heavy objects. And there is nothing wrong with that. However, we do not intentionally want to restrict the flow from an *Āyurvedic* perspective when menstruating.

Although the pelvic diaphragm is another subject, it is still important to mention here. Many people have a tight pelvic floor due to their posture and from being tense in general. Slouching on the sofa or in front of the computer tightens the pelvic floor muscles. It might also be very contracted if you strongly engage the pelvic floor through your yoga practice, exercise regime or because you are stressed or anxious. It is tight but not necessarily flexible or strong. Perhaps it is time to learn to relax and release the pelvic floor. If you want to focus on the pelvic floor during menstruation, you could teach students to relax and breathe into the pelvis rather than lifting and engaging.

- Don't practise *prāṇayāma* – manipulating the *prāṇa.*

Let's come back to *apāna vāyu*. It is one of the things we may manipulate or direct in our meditation practice and of course, in *prāṇayāma*, our breathing practices. Will this affect menstruation? Yes and no. If the focus is to manipulate and direct *prāṇa*, and to work with *mūlabandha* as described above, then yes. If we manipulate the flow of *prāṇa* we inadvertently also affect *apāna vāyu* and with that the action of menstruation.

But not all breathing practices or *prāṇayāma* have that intention. In fact, I find that attention to my breath helps enormously if I am experiencing strong sensations when I am on my period.

I wouldn't go for any forceful practices such as *kapālabhāti* (skull-shining breath) or *bhastrikā* (bellows breath) due to their impact on the lower abdomen or other variations where there is a specific focus on moving energy. But gentle *ujjâyî prāṇayāma* while seated or rocking, the *brāmari prāṇayāma* (bumblebee breath) or simply just slow diaphragmatic breathing are ways to release tension in the body and mind during cramps, discomfort and mental agitation.

- Don't manipulate *prāṇa* – meditation and devotional practice.

Meditation is so many things and in a general class for the general person, I can see no reason why a menstruating person shouldn't meditate. There are some considerations, though, depending on the meditation practice. Finding stillness, contemplating and retreating may be a natural inclination for many during the menstrual phase.

In some cultures, it is forbidden to go to the temple to pray and engage in devotional practices during menstruation. Often seen as a patriarchal restriction (and perhaps used as such for a long time and still is), this has its origin in the power of the menstrual energy. The temple is a place to encourage energy to rise, as we discussed in the section on cultural context, myths and wisdom in Chapter 4. We practise some meditation techniques and rituals for *apāna vāyu* to rise to meet *prāṇa vāyu*. That is not what we want during the menses where the downward flow of *apāna vāyu* is active. If *apāna vāyu* is imbalanced, *vāta doṣa* is imbalanced and it can be the beginning of an avalanche of *doṣic* issues.

We discussed *raktamokṣa*, or bloodletting, in the *Āyurveda* physiology section. Bloodletting is a way to relieve vitiated or imbalanced *rakta*, blood tissue, or *pitta* from blood. As the period is a natural occurrence of this process, we are resting and releasing. It may feel natural for us to contemplate and retreat, which in itself is also a spiritual practice and it is prompted naturally through the menstrual cycle. There is no need to manipulate our *prāṇa* or energy with specific practices.

- You should only rest on your period.

You may also have been told that rest is best on your period. Simply doing nothing at all. No yoga or exercise. The reason is the same as above: to rest during the special time when *apāna vāyu* needs no disturbance, and, perhaps more specifically, to rest as menstruation is nature's way of *raktamokṣa*, or bloodletting, as discussed above.

However, as busy people with work, activities, families and so on, we might not be able to create time to rest and do nothing. In fact, we might feel the need to move, be active and release some energy.

It's all about balance. *Āyurveda* teaches us to listen to our own bodies. As yoga teachers, we can encourage our students to check in with their bodies and their energy and notice what is right for them at that specific time. We should do the same for ourselves.

One research review and analysis (McNulty *et al.* 2020) concluded that 'exercise performance might be trivially reduced during the early follicular phase' (meaning the menstrual phase in medical language), but the study also confirmed that studies on this subject are sparse and generally poor quality at present.

Personally, as a yoga teacher, an *Āyurvedic* practitioner and menstruating person, I swing between just wanting to lie on the couch, wanting to do some *yin*-style relaxing restorative practice and sometimes really enjoying a *vinyāsa* flow towards the end of my menstrual phase. Sometimes my activity may be a simple walk in nature.

This does not just relate to our yoga *āsana* practice. Yoga and *Āyurveda* are about how we live our life. So if you had particularly stressful and physically tiring follicular and luteal phases then you might be completely drained and exhausted during the menstrual phase. But if the month has been supported and balanced, you may feel more energized and stronger during your period.

New research and lack of research

There is definitely a gender bias when it comes to medical research, including sports science. For example, in a review by Costello, Bieuzen and Bleackly (2012, p.847), 'Data were extracted from 1382 articles involving a total of 6,076,580 participants. A total of 2,366,968 (39%) participants were female and 3,709,612 (61%) were male.' The review concluded that, 'Females were significantly under-represented across all of the journals.' Another analysis (Cowley *et al.* 2021) concluded that 'women account for only 34% of the absolute number of participants included' and 'only 6% of total publications were conducted exclusively on women'.

Many more reviews and studies are highlighting this gender bias across medical science and research in general.

When we (or the researchers) don't consider how the different phases of the menstrual cycle and the changing hormones affect exercise, sports, surgery or medication, we lose out. The science becomes inconsistent due to how we can interpret the data. This can lead to 'potentially negative consequences for all individuals' as Steinberg *et al.* (2021) conclude in their analysis.

There are quite a few research papers on yoga and the menstrual cycle though. These mostly look at yoga programmes for either dysmenorrhea (painful periods) or premenstrual tension, and mental and emotional well-being and therefore quality of life. The quality of these research papers varies. There are so many factors involved when it comes to exercise, especially yoga as practised not just as *āsana* but also with a spiritual component. Having said that, the research does look very promising.

I will refer to relevant research as we move into the next chapters and as we explore specific complaints during the menstrual cycle.

CHAPTER 11

Practical Application of *Āyurvedic* Principles in Yoga

Now comes the practical and maybe more exciting bit. This chapter and the next ones are all about how to implement the knowledge and teachings you have learned so far. Here we are looking at how to teach and practise yoga according to the hormonal cycle and the *doṣic* changes. Then we will look at some of the specific complaints around the cycle we might encounter such as PMS and painful periods.

But first let's look at bringing our *Āyurvedic* principles and yoga practice together.

Regardless of what style or lineage of yoga you teach, you can personalize your teaching according to your students and clients. Just like you enquire regarding injuries, surgery or other health checks, you may start to ask about their cycle. In the sports world, we have coaches tailoring exercise programmes according to the athletes' cycles and hormones. I am aware that some people do not want to discuss periods at all. But many are starting to understand the benefits of doing so.

As yoga teachers, we can do the same. *Āyurveda* has clear principles on how to live according to the changing seasons and our unique constitution. This includes the changing phases during the menstrual cycle.

Here are a few points to remember from the introduction to *Āyurveda* and the *Āyurvedic* physiology sections.

> We all have a unique constitution. Our *prakṛti* is how we were born. We are unique individuals with unique needs and expressions. You may be mostly *pitta*, with some *vāta* and less *kapha*. And your student might be very *kapha*, with some *pitta* but little *vāta*. That is the natural state for the individual. Therefore, what works for one person may not be appropriate for another.

We are changing throughout our life. Our work situation, where we live, diet, lifestyle and life experiences all affect us. These factors create alterations to our *prakṛti*, which means we form what we call *vikṛti*. This is our current state. To find balance we want to restore our *prakṛti*.

During our lifespan as well as during the monthly cycle the *doṣas* will influence us. Childhood is dominated by *kapha*, as adults/in mid-life we are more *pitta* and later in life, it's natural to be influenced by *vāta*.

In the menstrual cycle, *vāta* is the instigator of menstruation, *kapha* of the follicular phase and *pitta* the luteal phase.

Shifting the focus in public classes

In a private or one-to-one yoga setting, we can tailor the experience to the individual and their unique situation. In a class setting, we acknowledge that everybody is an individual. Not everyone will have a menstrual cycle and those who do won't be in sync. So you will teach a class with people in their follicular phase, some menstruating and some in their luteal phase. Some have never had a menstrual cycle, some have but no longer do and some are taking hormones so may have breakthrough bleeds but no hormonal cycle or periods.

It may seem a complicated scenario but it doesn't need to be. In a yoga setting, we can offer options, modifications and adaptations of various poses. It does add an extra dimension when we include the menstrual cycle. But, in the end, it's about education and encouraging our students to listen to their bodies and energy.

We can educate our students about the hormonal and *doṣic* changes, letting them know how these may affect them physically and emotionally through the month. We can encourage self-awareness, learning to listen to the body and shifts in energy, perhaps suggesting tracking the menstrual cycle to notice patterns during the month. We can advise them to be aware of when the ego kicks in or perhaps when their *tāmasic* or *rajasic* tendencies of respectively being a little lazy and heavy or pushing themselves excessively are more prominent.

Relating this information to the phases of the moon gives everybody the potential to adjust. The actual moon phases can offer a framework that all of us can work with. We may associate the waxing moon with the follicular phase where we encourage a stronger more dynamic yoga. But a menstruating person can still adjust the practice and their intention for the class to go more inward or be more gentle if desired.

I generally set the mood for each class and offer options. If anyone is feeling fatigued I give options, encouraging them to let the practice be nourishing and nurturing. If the students have awareness of the menstrual cycle they might feel tired during their late luteal or menstrual phase. Maybe they can rest in a *bālāsana* (child's pose) or stay in *adhomukhaśvānāsana* (downward-facing dog) where those more energized can move through their connecting *vinyāsa* of plank pose, *chaturaṅgadaṇḍāsana* and *ūrdhvamukhaśvānāsana* (upward-facing dog). There are always options.

People in the follicular phase and during ovulation may feel more adventurous, have stronger stamina and have better muscular recovery. Those feeling strong and motivated can embrace the strengthening and dynamic aspects of the session. We can suggest a different and more challenging variation of a yoga pose, get into the alignment of the *āsana* or focus on muscular actions.

In open classes, I generally share options for those menstruating. These are not prescriptive, just options. If they really want to do *sālamba-sarvāṅgāsana* (shoulderstand) it's their choice. But I always offer the option of *viparīta karaṇī* (legs-up-the-wall). If it feels more appropriate to simply breathe complete diaphragmatic breathing rather than *kapālabhāti*, they will have that option. A more contemplative practice might also be appropriate during the dark moon.

With this framework in mind, we will go into more detail for each phase of the menstrual cycle and what *āsana* and intention we can bring to class.

Teaching *Āyurvedic* and cycle-aware yoga

Teaching group classes or public classes

Although group classes are general, we can educate students and discuss some of the concepts in this book. We can share how each student can check in with their own body, and where they are in their cycle, so they can adjust and modify their practice accordingly. It is very valuable information that is simple to introduce in a group setting or perhaps in a workshop. This could lead to menstrual-health-themed yoga classes, womb yoga and fertility yoga classes centring on how a healthy cycle is essential for fertility and therefore our general wellbeing, whether or not a person is trying to conceive.

Teaching from an *Āyurvedic* perspective we also take into account the external conditions such as the weather, seasons and environment. Living in the countryside is very different from living in a busy city. Is it a *pitta*-increasing hot humid summer day around lunchtime? A *vāta*-prevalent windy, dry and cold afternoon? Or a cold wet winter morning with *kapha* qualities?

We take all of these aspects of life into account when we teach our clients. We don't have to make it complicated. Most of it is intuitive. If it is a cold day we want to warm up. If our students are often travelling, living in the hustle and bustle of a big city, and we teach them during their workday in a busy office, we can encourage a calm and grounded practice.

One-to-one or private yoga sessions

It becomes even more interesting when we teach one-to-one. In a one-to-one session, we work directly with the person in front of us, their cycle and cyclic changes. We can invite them to embrace menstrual cycle awareness by tracking their cycle, writing notes on how they feel emotionally and mentally, how their body changes and any menstrual or premenstrual symptoms they may experience. They don't need to share it all with us. It's a way for them to understand their own body. Numerous apps are available to track the menstrual cycle and symptoms too.

When we, and they, understand how they feel at different phases of the cycle we can work *with* their body rather than *against* their physiology.

If you already teach one-to-one, this is just another dimension of how you look at your student as an individual and work with their body and their practice.

If you are teaching private sessions you may want to consider the following:

Why does the client want a private yoga session? They may have an injury they want to heal or perhaps a medical condition and they want a yoga practice that can support them along with their treatment. Perhaps they just like the individual attention and understand the value of working privately with an instructor. It may be convenient as they can have a yoga class at a time and place that works with their schedule rather than a studio timetable.

If you specialize and promote yourself as someone working with menstrual wellbeing, fertility, womb yoga or what is often referred to as women's yoga or women's health then you are growing the way you can support and tailor the yoga practice for your clients. You can truly work with them around their physiology, *doṣic* and energetically changing phases of the month. They may come to you specifically to support their fertility journey and that means a healthy cycle. Perhaps they present with severe PMS or menstrual cramps. You can use the tools and support you are learning in this book to create an individualized yoga programme for these private clients.

Your private client's aim and focus may very well have nothing to do with menstrual cycle awareness, period pains, PMS or fertility. Even if it isn't anything to do with their cycle I hope you recognize how much our hormones and *doṣas* affect our body, mind and yoga practice. Why not work *with* our physiology rather than *against* it or simply ignore it? Even if someone says they don't feel any different at any time during the month, you can still take advantage of the physiological changes.

Being an ever-evolving teacher or guide

The most important thing when it comes to *Āyurveda* and menstrual cycle awareness is to observe what works for the individual. The best person to notice, experience and navigate these shifts is the person themselves. We, as yoga teachers, can guide and support through our experience, research and training. We are not here to diagnose, heal or treat.

We have to learn to observe without judgement and preconceived ideas. That is what we are learning in yoga and *Āyurveda* – as yoga teachers and students.

Depending on your teaching style and how you work with private clients or in a therapeutic setting, you may take a detailed client history. Make notes after or during every session. Give the client sequences or poses to practise by themselves between your sessions.

As teachers, we also evolve our individual teaching style and teaching approach. What I am sharing here is simply another aspect of deepening or contemplating how you teach, regardless of whether you are more of a *yin*-style, dynamic flow, restorative or 'traditional' *haṭha* yoga teacher of any lineage.

I have found that students find it challenging to do homework, so I keep it very simple. I tend to offer things they can implement in their daily life: maybe some breathing or meditation they can do before they get out of bed; a stretch they can fit into a busy day at the office; a yoga pose variation they can practise while watching Netflix. No, it isn't ideal. But it is better than nothing. You may also have a sharp, determined *pitta* client who wants you to create an hour-long home practice they can do every day of the week. I find that shorter sequences or just a few poses work better for compliance. In the actual private yoga session, you can then truly focus and tune into what they need at the time.

Class planning according to the phases of the menstrual cycle

When you plan yoga classes or homework (if you give them sequences to do on their own) adjust it to their cycle. Here is a preview of what we will explore in the next few chapters.

Menstrual phase

Some students might just want to rest and do nothing, which is absolutely fine. Some may want a very restorative session, perhaps focusing on relieving symptoms such as cramps or heaviness.

Although *Āyurveda* would traditionally say this is a time of rest so as not to disturb *apāna vāyu*, some people feel energized, focused and determined to move. Consider the flow of *prāṇa* and avoid inversions and poses that require *mūlabandha*. Having said that, from a Western medical view there is no reason not to do inversions and our students choose how they prefer to move and practise.

Follicular phase (just after their period/end of period)

This is the best time to focus on strength, building muscle, trying new or more advanced or challenging poses. Dynamic flows and creative *vinyāsa* sequences are perfect now.

Ovulation phase

As in the follicular phase, there is energy and power at this time to explore and be creative.

Luteal phase

Although our menstrual health awareness is holistic and reflects the whole monthly cycle, this is a good time to check in with any PMS and menstrual complaints and address them now. The beginning of this phase is still excellent for power and strength but then the energy wanes. It is time to consider technique and alignment instead. This can also be a time when coordination becomes more challenging, which is worth keeping in mind if you like creative flow sequences. The body temperature, and *pitta doṣa*, rises and your client might feel hot and sweaty sooner than usual.

Exercise according to *Āyurveda*

Exercise is part of our general health and wellbeing. According to *Caraka*, one of the classic teachers of *Āyurveda*, exercise creates stability and strength and has to be practised in moderation. It brings lightness, ability to work (as it increases fitness levels) and also supports digestion.

Resistance to discomfort

One of the benefits of exercise, according to *Caraka*, is that it gives resistance to discomfort. As a yoga teacher, I find this interesting. Yoga is not always comfortable. For example, some of us find plank pose extremely challenging. But as we practise it and become stronger or perhaps understand the shape better, we increase that resistance to discomfort. Or perhaps you resist deep stretches such as *kapotāsana* (pigeon pose). Some people love it and others experience discomfort and resistance. What about deep backbends like *dhanurāsana* (wheel pose)? Maybe the discomfort is physical yet we may be within our abilities of mobility and strength to do it. Perhaps it is the mental resistance to the *āsana* that causes discomfort.

Yoga is such a great tool to explore resistance, especially mental resistance and discomfort beyond the yoga class. This is where we can integrate the teachings of yoga into how we navigate resistance, discomfort and challenges in our daily life off the mat.

In the *Caraka-saṃhitā Sutrasthana* it says that exercise can alleviate the *doṣas*, especially *kapha. Kapha doṣa* can be stagnant, slow and solid. Exercise is the perfect way to decrease excess *kapha.*

But can you have too much of a good thing?

Anything in excess is never a good thing. Indeed, *Caraka* explains how excessive exercise can lead to exertion, exhaustion, consumption, thirst as well as bleeding, cough, fever and vomiting.

He continues to explain that 'one who indulges in...excess [exercise] suddenly perishes like a lion trying to drag a huge elephant'. This warns that you can perish, or die, from exhaustion. Any movement is *vāta*. Excess exercise and movement can increase *vāta. Pitta* may increase due to heat and perspiration. In turn, the heat of *pitta doṣa* can cause dryness, which leads to further *vāta* aggravation. In excess, this is detrimental to our health and wellbeing.

From an *Āyurvedic* perspective, if we are prone to increased *vāta* or *pitta* we need to be mindful of how we exercise, especially during the luteal or premenstrual phases where *pitta* is likely to be aggravated, and during menstruation where *vāta* is already increased. Yoga is excellent because we can adjust and focus on what we need at any given time.

The *Āyurvedic* classics explain that correct exercise gives just the right amount of perspiration (a light sweat on the forehead, armpits and spine), enhances respiration, creates a lightness of the body and supports the heart and other organs.

Exercise and movement are essential according to *Āyurveda* – but in balance.

Pitta needs less heat and power. Instead, favour calming and cooling practices, both for the body and the mind.

Vāta is already light and mobile so needs more stillness, strength and stability in body and mind.

Kapha needs to increase mobility, active movement and warmth, as it has slow and dull tendencies.

Creating doṣic balance with yoga

We often say that a balanced person will know exactly what they need to stay in equilibrium. But when we are slightly out of balance we are often drawn to what we already have too much of. You will see this tendency in your students too and will most likely have observed it within yourself.

An imbalanced *pitta* person who is already hot, irritable and highly strung will often seek out a hot power yoga class, which would increase *pitta* even further. However, a slow flow yoga class, or gentle movement with some *yin*, restorative or meditative practice would balance out the excess heat and hot, sharp temperament.

An imbalanced *vāta* person who is already fidgety, a little spaced out and ungrounded might be drawn to a more esoteric *kuṇḍalinī* yoga (in the Yogi Bhajan style) or a dynamic creative *vinyāsa* flow class. The *kuṇḍalinī* class will increase the space and air elements making a *vāta* person even more ungrounded and potentially anxious. However, the *vinyāsa* class can be perfect to get into the body rather than being in the head. But the *vāta* person needs to keep the flow grounded and focused, rather than bouncy or jumpy. This can also be achieved with a slow meditative flow, traditional *haṭha* yoga or an alignment-based class where there is focus on the body such as Iyengar-style yoga or a restorative or *yin*-style class.

People with excess and vitiated *kapha* might not want to move at all, not wanting to attend any sort of movement or yoga class except a sound bath or yoga *nidra*. Both are great for everybody and any *doṣa*. But if there is an excess of stagnant, heavy and slow *kapha*, it needs to be balanced. A dynamic flow class and plenty of sun salutations are excellent for *kapha*. Because *kapha* can accumulate in the lungs and chest, *prāṇayāma* practices are also highly recommended.

Obesity, body types and overdoing it

We may be living in a culture where type-A personalities, ambition and being busy are celebrated. Even our children are encouraged to attend a full weekly calendar of activities. But according to *Āyurveda*, it just isn't helpful for our health.

Much of our exercise is doing more, pushing ourselves, gaining more, sweating more. Even in the yoga environment, people turn up with injuries because of striving to be better, fitter. It is all very *pitta*.

Yet we also have an obesity epidemic where one in four adults and one in every five children between 10 and 11 years old in the UK are obese, according to the NHS (National Health Service 2019). It isn't just imbalanced *kapha* types who are obese because of feeling slow, heavy or low. Anyone can have an unhealthy weight for their individual constitution. Yoga and *Āyurveda* are such great techniques to create an environment for finding balance within the individual. It's not only about physical exercise or a diet plan. It is about the individual, physically, mentally, emotionally and spiritually. In yoga, we can also consider the qualities of *sattva*, *rajas* and *tāmas*. A *tāmasic* attitude can lead to laziness, heaviness and feeling low. This in turn could lead to non-activity, which can lead a person to eat excessively or have no interest in food at all. Neither is healthy. And that is what we, as yoga teachers, need to appreciate when we teach our students and create our yoga classes.

Understanding body types

You may have heard about the body types or classifications of endomorph, mesomorph and ectomorph. Endomorphs have more muscle mass, fat and curves, a mesomorph has a more athletic build and ectomorphs are generally long and lean. In *Āyurveda*, we can compare them with the *doṣic* body types:

Kapha people of water and earth appear solid, more curvaceous and tend to gain weight and body fat easily similar to endomorphs.

Pitta people with plenty of fire element have an athletic build and can gain muscle and definition easily just like mesomorphs. Weight is reasonably stable.

Vāta people, being influenced by air and space, are light and slim just like ectomorphs. They find it challenging to put on weight.

As always, remember that we are all a combination of the three *doṣas* and five elements. A *vāta*-dominant person can also gain weight and a *kapha* person can be very slender.

Mental and physical wellbeing and the benefits of yoga

Mental health, depression and anxiety are significant problems in our community. According to the UK charity Mind (2020), one in four people will experience a mental health issue each year in the UK and one in six reports experiencing a common mental health issue such as anxiety and depression in any given week in England. There are, of course, numerous reasons but certainly stress and anxiety of daily life, how we are expected to live and look as well as work-related pressure are part of those reasons. We know stress affects our hormones and therefore also the menstrual cycle, just as our relationship to the cycle affects our emotional wellbeing too.

Yoga is a tool to support our mental and emotional health, through the physical *āsana* or regular yoga classes as well as the philosophy and spiritual teachings of yoga. And so is *Āyurveda.*

Researching peer-reviewed medical journals, I found plenty of evidence of the many physical and emotional benefits of yoga. This was the topic of my dissertation for my BSc (Bachelor of Science) in *Āyurveda* (Lange 2009). Since then, even more studies have come out confirming the positive outcomes of practising yoga. We have most likely experienced those benefits ourselves too – and we have witnessed them in our yoga students.

Yet, we also know that no approach works for everybody every time. We have to adjust to our particular *doṣic* makeup and to our environment, including where we are in our menstrual cycle.

Once again, we need to look at and teach to the individual. When we work with our clients or students on menstrual awareness for their yoga practice, we also need to take into account how they approach exercise. Is it with the determination and focus of *pitta*, the playfulness and sometimes scatterbrained characteristics of *vāta* or the potentially unmotivated style of *kapha* who, in fact, has lots of stamina and endurance?

Most importantly, this is their practice and their experience. Yoga and *Āyurveda* are ways to understand our body and mind. We can encourage our students to take responsibility, track their cycle, connect with their body, emotions and mental tendencies – and we have to learn to be the observer and guide.

CHAPTER 12

Yoga for Each Phase of the Menstrual Cycle

Menstrual cycle versus menstrual phase

It is important to recognize that menstruation is a vital sign of our general health. If there are any imbalances such as pain, clotting, heavy periods, extreme tiredness or no menstruation at all, it is a sign that something is off. Menstruation is a brilliant guide for our general health and wellbeing.

The menstrual cycle is a full cycle, not just the bleeding time. We experience most complaints at the menstrual phase but any imbalance will have been there throughout the cycle and may just manifest during the bleed. Indeed, many research papers on the effect of yoga on menstrual complaints incorporate yoga practices throughout the month, not just during the menstrual phase.

Yoga during the menstrual phase

Day 1 of the menstrual cycle is the first day of bleeding. This does not include spotting, but is when the menstruation begins properly. If we teach yoga students who are not menstruating, we can equate this with the dark or new moon transition.

As a reminder, this is when our hormones are at their lowest. Because of the low hormones, some (but not all) people feel incredibly tired and fatigued at this time.

Prostaglandins are released. These are hormone-like chemicals that can cause inflammation, pain and sometimes diarrhoea. Because of these symptoms and loss of energy, some people simply want to enjoy the menstrual phase as a time for introspection, rest and recovery.

Having said that, other people thrive on this low hormone phase. They feel more like themselves without the hormones clouding their vision or connection to their body and mind.

It is important to remember that we are all unique. Allow each individual to notice how this phase affects them.

In the chapter on *Āyurvedic* physiology, we discussed how important the menstrual phase is. Here is a quick recap:

> *Apāna vāyu* is responsible for menstruation. It is the downward moving energy and a sub*doṣa* of *vāta*. From an *Āyurvedic* perspective, it is essential that *apāna vāyu* isn't disturbed during menstruation.
>
> *Raktamokṣa* is the cleansing process of purifying excess *rakta*, blood tissue, from the body. If we have increased *pitta doṣa*, it will often go to the blood tissue and *raktamokṣa* is the perfect way to clear excess *pitta* or *rakta*. This is what happens when we bleed. During any cleanse, we rest to allow the body to fulfil its natural processes.

What to avoid during the menstruation phase

As we discussed in the myths and facts section, it's important to allow everyone to make their own informed decisions and do their own research.

From a Western perspective, there is no reason not to practise inversions such as *śīrṣāsana* (headstand) or *adhomukhavṛkṣāsana* (handstand). There is no research exploring the effect of various meditations or breathing practises during menstruation. But Western medical research and science work on the *sthūlaśārira*, the gross and physical body. Those of us practising yoga rather than callisthenics, pilates, personal training or gymnastics may also take into account the *sūkṣmaśārira*, which is the subtle energetic body. Looking at it from an *Āyurvedic* perspective, appreciating the *sūkṣmaśārira*, the elements, the *vāyus* and *doṣas*, there are contraindications and modifications during the bleeding phase. To sum up what we discussed already, *Āyurveda* has some specific suggestions:

- No manipulation of *prāṇa*. Any breathing practices or meditations where you encourage *prāṇa* to rise are contraindicated from an energetic perspective as we do not want to disturb *apāna vāyu*.
- No inversions. This includes *sālambasarvāṅgāsana* (shoulderstand), *śīrṣāsana* (headstand), *piñchhamayūrāsana* (forearmstand) and *adhomukhavṛkṣāsana* (handstand). In these poses, you are inverting *apāna vāyu*, manipulating it in its opposite direction.

- No *bandhas. Bandhas*, or energetic seals or locks, are used specifically to manipulate *prāṇa* or energy in the body which we do not want to do during menstruation. This can be either energetically in meditation or physically in *āsana*. If we use *mūlabandha* as a way to engage and lift the pelvic floor it works similarly both physically and energetically. Although the pelvic diaphragm will engage and relax naturally as we move and breathe, we don't want to apply it with intention during this time.
- Avoid excess *apāna* through squats or similar *āsana*. Just as we don't want to manipulate *apāna vāyu* or *prāṇa* in general during menstruation through inversions or *bandhas*, we also don't want excess *apāna*. *Malāsana* (yogic squat) is one of the poses we generally associate with increasing *apāna vāyu*. It is recommended for other *apāna* actions such as easing bowel movements as well as modified variations at some stages in pregnancy and childbirth. However, during a balanced or heavy menstruation we do not want to encourage any excess *apāna* by squatting, or other *āsana* that may have the same energy.

From a Western hormonal perspective, there are no contraindications except to listen to your body, take an individual approach and allow for rest if you experience pain, dizziness, diarrhoea or a heavy bleed. It may be the perfect rest phase for your physical exercise regime.

What to encourage during the menstrual phase

In Chapter 14, we go into detail about some of the common complaints during the menstrual phase and yoga poses that may be useful. It might simply be best to rest, especially if there is heavy bleeding or pain. Remember, rest is powerful. We need time to recover and slow down.

However, if there isn't any severe discomfort, moderate movement can increase endorphins, which are our feel-good hormones. This can include gentle exercise, yoga or walking.

The guṇas and the menstrual phase

From yoga and *Āyurveda* philosophy, we recognize the three *guṇas*: *sattva*, *rajas* and *tāmas*. Menstruation is called *rajahsrāva*. It is the time when *rajas guṇa* can leave the (subtle) body (*sūkṣmaśārira*) through the blood tissue. We can then either gravitate towards *tāmas* or *sattva*.

Tāmas is stagnation and inertia. *Tāmas* is lying down and feel sorry for ourselves, feeling depressed and experiencing dullness and lethargy.

Although we may feel tired and dull during menstruation, moving towards *sattva* is encouraged, finding ways to move with stillness and contemplative and mindful awareness. However you choose to approach yoga during the menstrual phase, it can be with this *sattvic* intention. We can encourage the feel-good endorphins and *sattva* rather than *tāmas* or *rajas*. It is the perfect time for inner reflection and contemplation, without getting drawn into the *tāmasic* heaviness.

Balance vāta doṣa

Vāta doṣa is dry, light, cold, rough, subtle, and is about movement. In a balanced body, this movement is associated with releasing the menstrual blood. During menstruation, we honour *vāta doṣa* and try not to disturb this with excess movement. *Vāta*-balancing yoga is anything that is warming, grounded and embodied. It is smooth and steady. If we move steadily, smoothly and slowly we honour the movement of *vāta* and avoid the heaviness of *tāmas*. Any erratic, quick or very sharp dynamic movement can aggravate both *vāta* and *pitta*.

Setting the mood for the yoga class during the menstrual phase

Everybody feels different during the menstrual phase. Many crave comfort, warmth and ease. These are natural cravings to balance *vāta doṣa*, which is cold, can be unstable, and is about mobility and lightness. We are all aiming to find balance. If you can, create a warm environment. You don't want it hot as this can aggravate *pitta* and any excess heat or *rakta* in the blood tissue. Heat can also dry out the already dry qualities of *vāta doṣa*.

It's the perfect time for more restorative yoga where you hold the poses for longer. It is good to use props, bolsters, sandbags, cushions and blankets.

You may also want to use a steady calm voice as a yoga instructor. Sound is associated with the element of space, which is part of *vāta doṣa*. Using your voice to slow down, ground and calm *vāta* is another way to support your menstruating students. If you use music in the classes, *vāta*-reducing beats would be slow, steady and low. Downtempo dub, classical Indian music (such as *ragas*), drums, deep or soothing sounds could all feature on your playlist.

Dimmed lights or candles (electric or real if possible) can calm an overactive *vāta* mind and create a comforting, warm and nurturing environment.

Intentions during the menstrual cycle

Remember that these are the first few days of a new cycle – either of the menstrual cycle or moon cycle. It is time to acknowledge what we are releasing along with the blood. What are we letting go of? What is no longer needed? What are we holding on to that is ready to be released?

For example, in *Āyurveda*, excess heat, fire, *rajasic* tendencies or *pitta doṣa* may be released through the blood as *rakta dhātu*, the blood tissue. This is what makes us boil over, burn out or show irritability and anger (all *pitta* qualities). We can consider letting go of anything that no longer serves us.

Once we let go, what are we creating space for? What are we inviting in for the next cycle? What seeds or intentions are we planting for the new monthly, lunar or moon cycle? What do we want to grow as the moon waxes for the new moon cycle?

Let's practise some yoga

According to *Āyurveda*, the menstrual phase shouldn't be painful. In a balanced person, we may notice the changes in energy but there should be no specific complaints. In this section, we focus on the healthy, balanced cycle, yet acknowledge some of the common complaints. When you read Chapter 14 on yoga for specific complaints, you can also implement those suggestions in your classes or private sessions.

The menstrual phase could be the perfect time to embrace the variations of *chandranāmaskar*, the moon salutation. Practise this with intention and a connection with the moon and its nourishing cooling energy. *Chandranāmaskar* can also be practised as a moving meditation. This offers a steady regular movement for *vāta doṣa* and focuses any nervous energy in both body and mind. It also cools down excess *pitta* yet stimulates any heavy stagnant *kapha*. Any slow flow or steady regular meditative movement can do the same.

Yin or restorative-style yoga is perfect for balancing *vāta* and supporting the body during the menstrual phase. Staying in one position for a while can help any scattered *vāta* energy to calm down and become grounded. Feeling anxious, nervous and experiencing insomnia can be excess *vāta doṣa* manifesting during menses. Being in a still and stable yoga pose, perhaps with plenty of support using cushions, bolsters, blocks or belts, will help balance *vāta doṣa*.

Hip openers and leg stretches complement *apāna vāyu* during the menstrual phase. *Apāna vāyu* and *vāta doṣa* are associated with the pelvis and the legs. Creating space and focusing the energy in the pelvic area during the *āsana* practice can support *apāna vāyu*, though not increase it or reverse it. I do not recommend *malāsana* (yogīc squats) or similar poses during menses as this can increase *apāna* and potentially cause heavier menstruation.

It is a good time to allow the abdomen to relax and soften. *Shavāsana* and yoga *nidra* both calm the mind and are nourishing for *vāta doṣa*. If someone doesn't feel like being mobile, these practices can be a perfect way to enjoy yoga without any movement.

Āsana and sequencing

Let's remind ourselves that we are all individuals and completely unique beings. That is true in *Āyurveda* when it comes to the *doṣas* and our *prakṛti* (constitution) as well as any imbalances manifesting as our *vikṛti*, current state. Maybe we have had a few well-balanced months with nourishing foods and good mental and emotional wellness. Perhaps we have been feeling stressed, drained or travelled a lot. Maybe our diet has suffered and we feel completely imbalanced. All of this will affect how we feel during the menstrual phase. The best thing is for the individual to track their cycle. This way we find a general pattern within all the variables.

If you, or your student, feel completely fatigued, perhaps in pain or have other complaints, the practice will be different compared to someone feeling really into their sacred empowered menstruation and having energy and strength. We cannot presume one or the other. Personally, I can feel great and enjoy most practices during my light to moderate bleed but if I experience more pain or a heavy flow, I don't feel like doing much. Where I might have enjoyed deep lunges or hip openers having a lighter bleed they are just not comfortable when I have a heavy flow. There is no right or wrong. Our yoga practice is up to how we feel at the time.

Sequencing

VIPARĪTA KARAṆĪ (LEGS-UP-THE-WALL)

Lying down with the legs up the wall or lower legs on a chair is a grounding and soothing practice for our nervous system. As we calm our nervous system, any excess *vāta doṣa* is also regulated. The nervous system and *vāta* are connected. *Viparīta karaṇī* (legs-up-the-wall) is not an inversion. The legs might be up but the energy of the legs, or femurs, is grounding and settling in the hip sockets. Remember, the pelvis is the seat of *vāta* and *apāna vāyu*, so rooting the energy here is perfect during menstruation – and at any time to settle disturbed *vāta*.

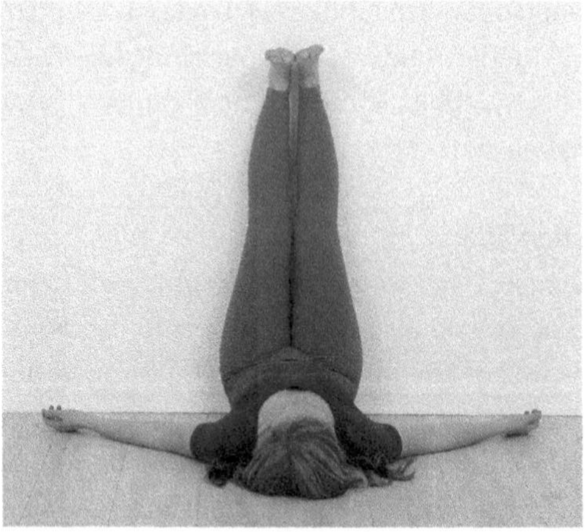

Viparīta karaṇī (legs-up-the-wall). Adjust so the back is neutral and the pelvis and back are comfortable. You can also place a bolster or sandbag onto the feet

HIP-OPENING POSE/FIGURE OF FOUR

Hip-opening against the wall. Crossing one ankle over the opposite knee as in a figure four position is another way to stay settled and grounded, connecting to both the floor and the wall. This also creates space in the pelvic area and opens any tightness around the hips, glutes and lower back, which can often feel restricted when menstruating.

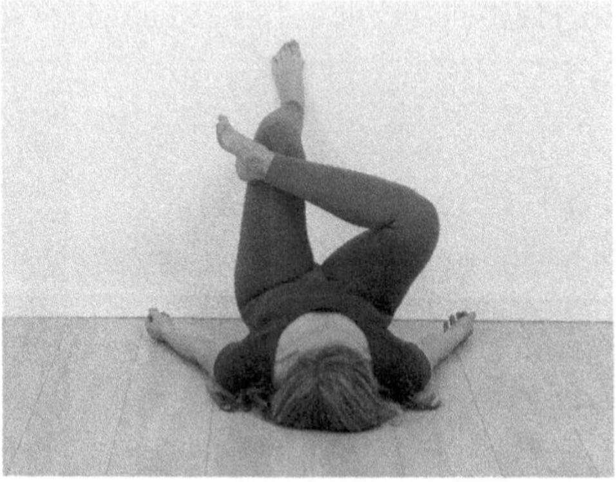

As in viparīta karaṇī, make sure the pelvis and back are comfortable as you cross the legs

SEATED MEDITATION/WELCOME

After the wall variations, I like to sit with the class or the private student to settle them, set intentions and welcome them to the practice. You may add a reading from a text, *mantra*, poem or chanting here as well.

UJJÂYÎ PRĀṆAYĀMA AND ROCKING

Ujjayi prāṇayāma is the meditative breath we feel and hear in the throat area. Breathing through the nose there is a gentle ocean sound in the throat. It can be a heating breath and *pitta* aggravating if done very loudly and with force, but if it comes naturally, like the sound of a baby sleeping or when entering into meditation, it can be very calming and soothing.

Adding a gentle natural rocking forwards and backwards with this meditative breath can be a wonderful way to create mobility and flow for both the blood and lymphatic circulation in the pelvic area. For me and many of my clients, this rocking has taken us through plenty of cramps and aches.

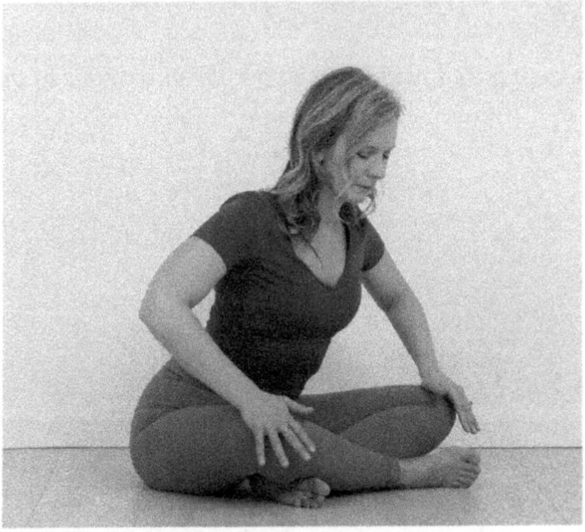

Pelvic rocking

BĀLĀSANA – CHILD'S POSE

Introducing *bālāsana* (child's pose) is a perfect start to the session. It also allows the students to return to this pose at any time in their practice when they feel the need for rest. *Bālāsana* helps to stretch the lower back and outer hips, the seat of *vāta doṣa* and *apāna vāyu* and a place where many experience pain during menstruation. When we have pain we often contract our body and the energy gets stagnant. Here you are trying to release and breathe.

If there are cramps or discomfort in the lower abdomen, we tend to fold naturally, either in the child's pose or a fetal position. If there is relief with pressure on the abdomen, students can make a double fist with their hands and place the fists just above the pubic bone as they fold forward into *bālāsana*.

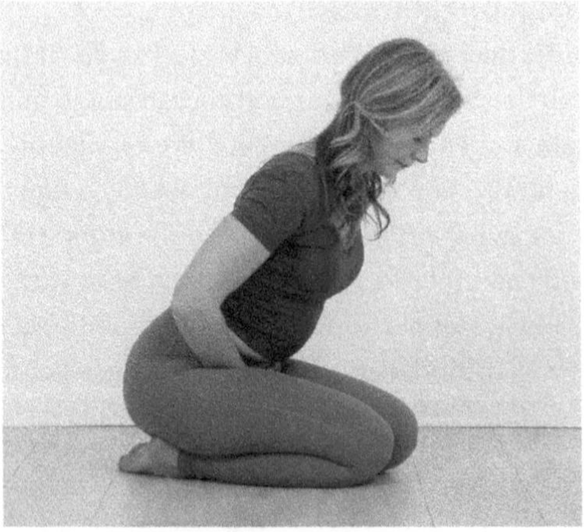

Make fists with the hands and place them above the pubic bone at the lower abdomen

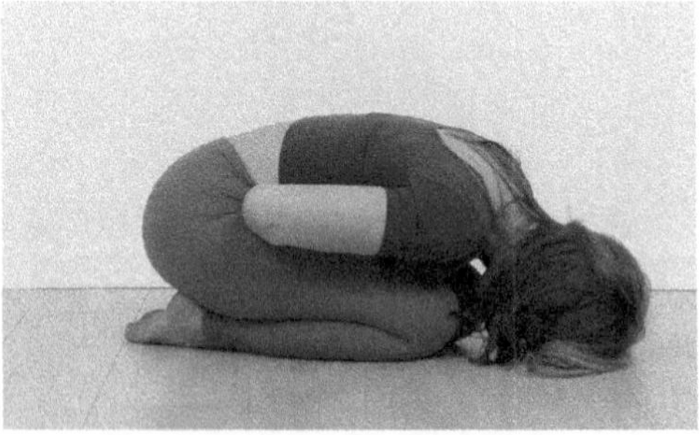

Fold over the fists and breathe deeply into the abdomen

As *vāta* is movement, light and feeling ungrounded, adding extra touch and support like the fists on the abdomen and being close to the mat or a bolster can bring relief. If you have bolsters you can also offer a *bālāsana* over the bolster.

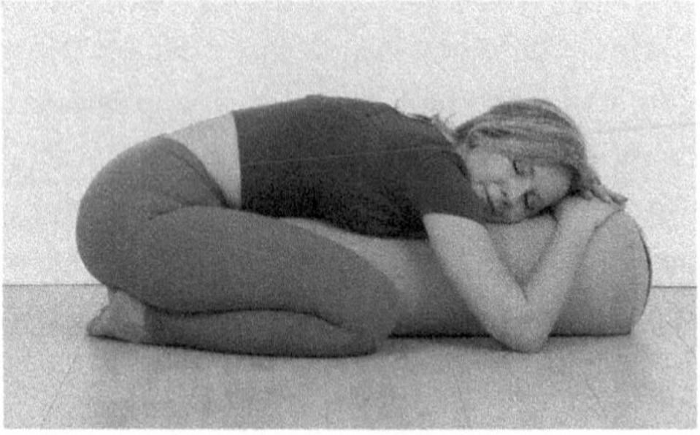

Bālāsana with a bolster

HANDS-AND-KNEES OR CAT-COW POSE

Any hands-and-knees positions can be a lovely fluid transition. They can be an alternative in a flow class instead of *adhomukhaśvānāsana* (downward-facing dog) or *chaturaṅgadaṇḍāsana* if your students prefer other options. Most of us know the cat-cow variation of flexing and extending the spine. This can bring release to muscular tension around the lower back and the pelvis. Rocking the pelvis in this way mobilizes and supports muscles around the pelvis, the pelvic floor, lower back as well as the fascia and ligaments connecting to the womb and ovaries.

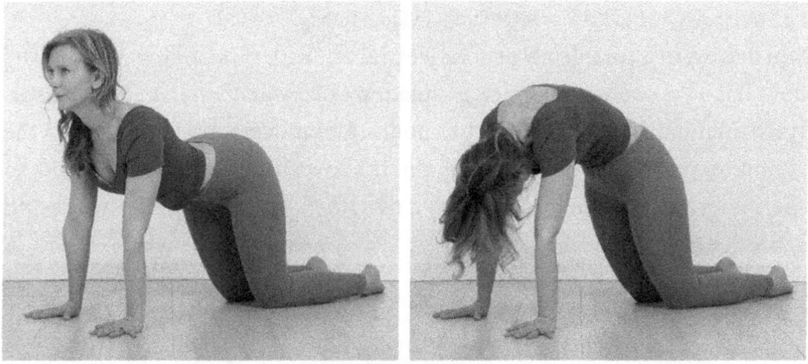

Moving in cat-cow pose

Hands-and-knees variations such as moving in circular or figure of eight shapes or any way the body wants to flow create an intuitive flow for our menstruating students. It can be gentle, meditative and sensual, or dynamic and focused, whatever the individual feels is appropriate. It allows us to explore what feels good in the body and adjust to what is needed at the time.

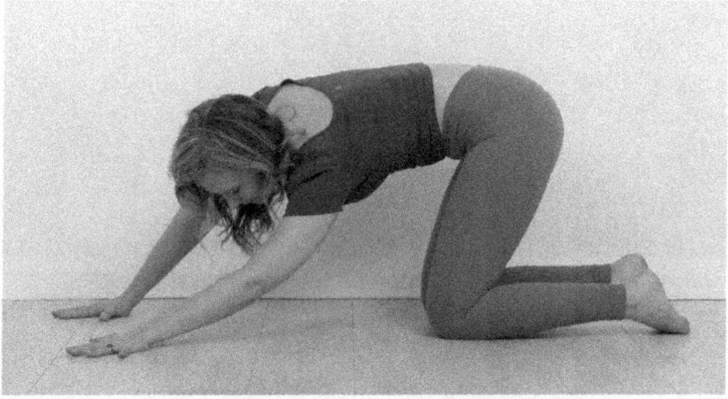

Intuitive fluid circular movements

ADHOMUKHAŚVĀNĀSANA – DOWNWARD-FACING DOG

You may wonder if this is an inversion or even a half inversion. Energetically, you are not extending all the energy up as if you were in a *śīrṣāsana* (headstand) or *sālambasarvāṅgāsana* (shoulderstand). Although the hips are high, you are rooting down through the legs and heels. In my felt and observed experience, *adhomukhaśvānāsana* is grounding and beneficial for the lower back pain, legs and any calf ache during menstruation. It provides a natural neutral spine, creates space at the pelvic floor and if one feels heavy pressure here it can offer some relief.

CHANDRANĀMASKAR – MOON SALUTATIONS

You may want a completely restorative practice with no standing poses or any flow. But if you were to embrace a salutation or *vinyāsa* then *chandranāmaskar* (moon salutation) is the perfect honouring of movement meditation to the changing phases of the moon. Again, it allows the individual to adjust to their energy. It can be practised in a dynamic way, or in a meditative and reflective way.

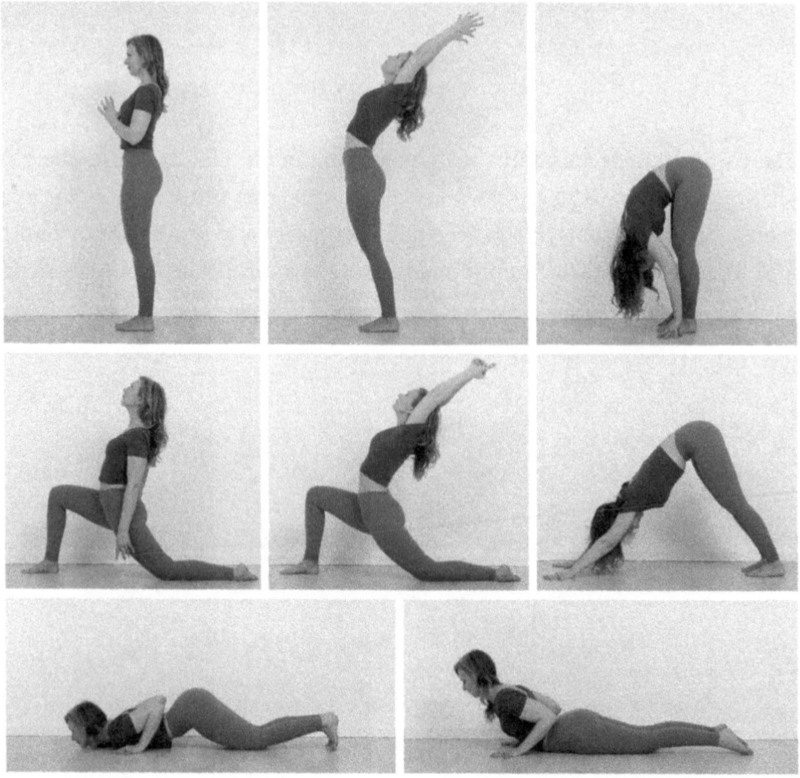

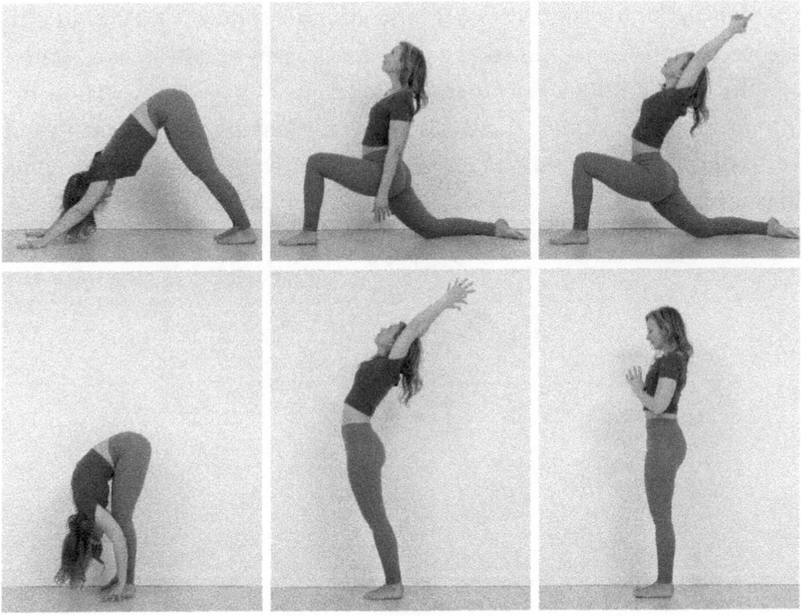

Chandranāmaskar is a sequence of 14 poses representing 14 phases of the moon

STANDING SEQUENCE

After our *sūryanamaskāra* (sun salutations), or in this instance *chandranāmaskar* (moon salutations), we often move into standing poses or a standing flow. Rather than suggesting specific poses here, it is worth remembering how we can change the focus and intention of the same yoga pose and experience it very differently. Indeed, you or your students might not want to do anything but lie on the floor with plenty of cushions, which is absolutely appropriate too. The first few days of the menstrual phase could be no yoga or no strong and standing poses at all. But after a few days, we may feel more energized and want to move again. This is about listening to our body and energy, not the ego.

We don't want to disturb *apāna vāyu* or aggravate *vāta* and *pitta doṣa* in the menstrual phase. We want the focus to be nourishing and nurturing to calm *vāta* and cool down any excess *pitta*. This may not be the time to hold a pose for an extra long time, go deeper or try a more 'advanced' variation. Perhaps choose a more fluid creative slow flow instead of a solar, alignment-based, hardcore, dynamic and quicker movement flow.

Most standing poses, including balancing poses, can be very meditative which is perfect at this time. We, as yoga teachers, can also offer contemplations relating to this time of the cycle. For example, as a warrior, in any of the *vīrabhadrāsana* (warrior pose) variations, what are we clearing out with the bleed and what are we creating space for as a new menstrual cycle starts?

The same question for *natarajāsana* (dancer's pose) as we dance the *Tāṇḍava*, the dance of life and destruction. What are we destroying and letting go of at this sacred time? And what are we embracing for this coming lunar cycle?

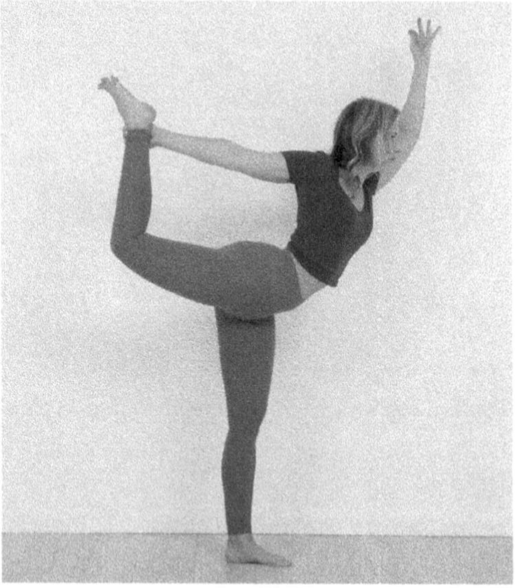

Natarajāsana

Balancing yet grounding poses such as *vrkāsana* (tree pose) may also feel appropriate, both as a hip-opening pose, balancing pose and as a pose where we are rooting into the earth. This can alleviate excess *vāta* and connect with *apāna vāyu.*

I'll add in standing forward bends here as well. Forward bends are said to calm the mind. An overactive mind is a sign of excess *vāta*. Bowing downwards and inwards can help us find balance and meditative contemplation. The forward bends may release constrictions and restrictions for the flow of *apāna vāyu. Apāna vāyu* needs to flow naturally and easily in the energetics of the pelvis and legs. Forward bends help as they extend the back of the legs, including the hamstrings and calf muscles, which can tighten during menses, as well as the lower back. The gentle compression of the lower abdomen may also offer relief from cramps and discomfort.

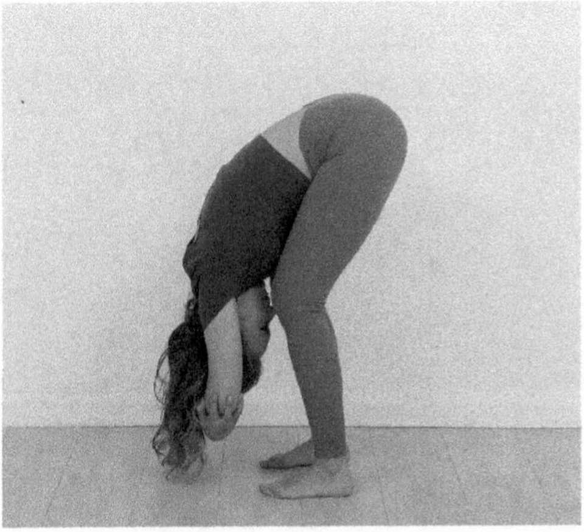

Standing forward bend with knees slightly bent holding on to the opposite elbows

FLOOR-BASED POSES

We will look at poses for specific complaints in detail in Chapter 14, where there are several floor-based poses. Let's consider some of the things we discourage. This includes stopping the flow of *apāna* such as using *mūlabandha*, tightening the pelvic floor, or doing inversions. We also don't want excess flow encouraged in poses such as *malāsana* or yogīc squats (except if you have an extremely light flow or only spotting). Instead, we encourage circulation of blood, *rakta dhātu*, and plasma or lymph, *rasa dhātu*, through our yoga practice. When we are in discomfort, we usually respond by tightening our muscles, including the pelvic floor, which restricts blood flow and, via the fascia and ligaments, might also affect the uterus and therefore the experience of intense sensations during menses.

Here are some of my favourite floor-based *yogāsana* to create ease around the pelvis. They comprise lower abdomen and hip flexor stretches, hip-openers with external rotation of the femur in the hip socket (acetabulum), and stretching the area around the sacrum, including the glutes and piriformis muscles:

- *Ustrāsana* (camel pose), which also gives lightness and is uplifting if one is feeling low and heavy.

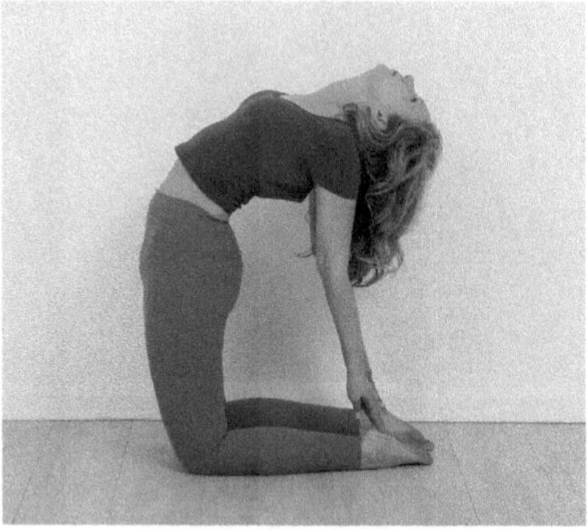

Ustrāsana can be adjusted to hold on to the sacrum or blocks, making sure the lower back isn't compressed

- *Setubandhāsana* (bridge pose) is an excellent pose to find openness in the front of the pelvis and hip flexors. It's a pose where you can offer some creativity and flow to allow your menstruating students ways to ease any tension around the sacrum and sacroiliac joints. *Setubandhāsana* can be very fluid and sensual too. Another option is to add support under the sacrum, as in a supported *setubandhāsana.*

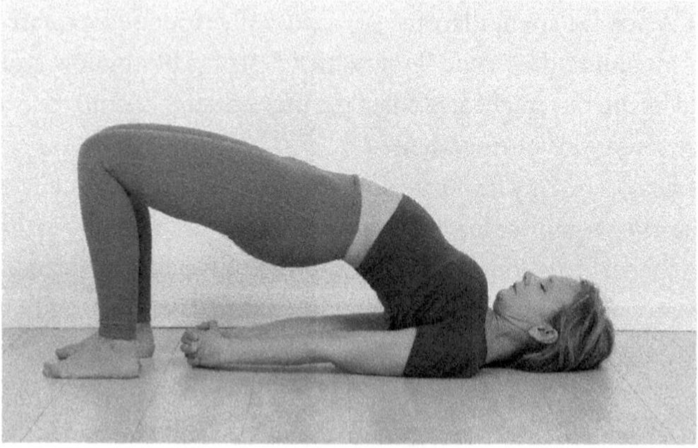

Setubandhāsana

- *Suptabaddhakonāsana* (reclined cobbler's pose) is perfect when supported with cushions or bolsters under the thighs.

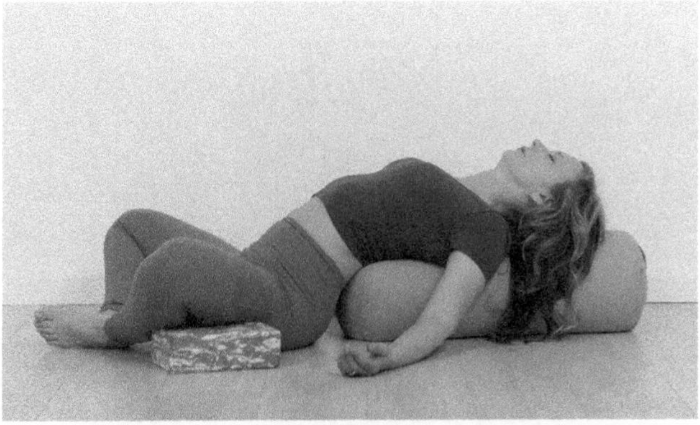

Suptabaddhakonāsana with optional bolster and blocks

- Seated forward bends are similar to the standing bends but are even more relaxed. Modify them and use props to make any forward bend appropriate for your students. We hinge from the hip joints rather than bending the lower back. If compression of the lower abdominal area gives pain relief, the student can add fists or a small rolled blanket just above the pubic bone as they hinge forward.

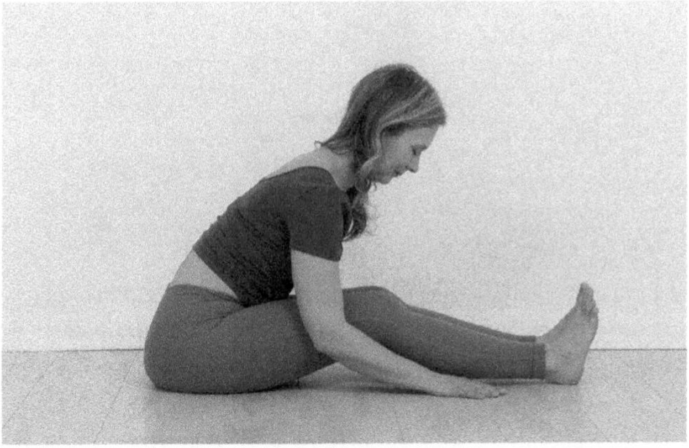

Modified seated forward bend

- Another option is folding forward in *gomukāsana* (cow pose) leg variation. The area around the sacrum, sacroiliac joints, piriformis and glutes is often tight and is a typical *vāta* ache. This position is a variation that releases tension and creates space, as do double pigeon or fire-log pose variations, where one lower leg is on top of the other. The actual *kapotāsana* (pigeon pose) also offers this kind of relief.

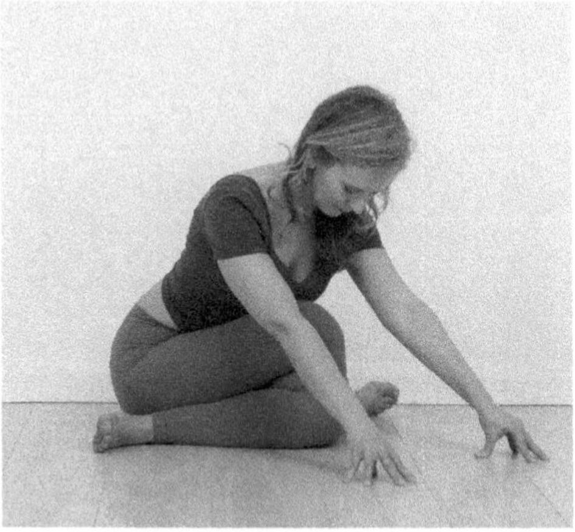

Gomukāsana variation. Modify by sitting upright on cushions or blocks

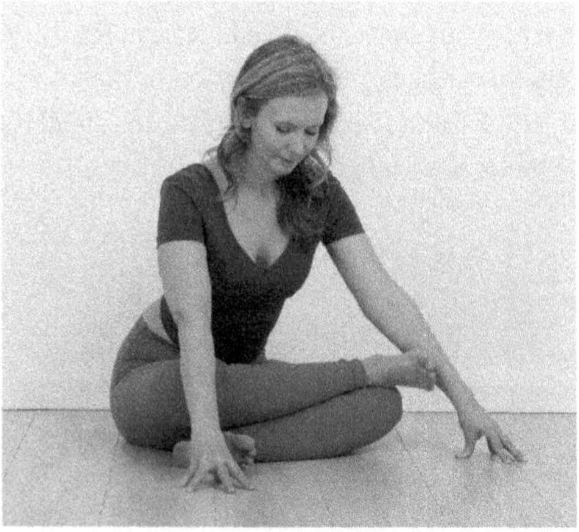

Placing the heel on top of the opposite knee and the other knee over the opposite foot. Add support where needed. Do not practise if there is any pain in the knee or hip joints

More importantly from an *Āyurvedic* perspective, all these poses can pacify excess *vāta doṣa*. They are grounding, static, slow and steady, and we can stay in these poses for a while and focus on the breath. This will help to soothe the nervous system and can provide pain relief. Remember, *vāta doṣa* is associated with the nervous system as well as pain.

Resting and meditation

Although we don't want to disturb the *prāṇa* or *vāyu* during menstruation we can still enjoy mindful breathing and slowing down. Yoga *nidra* is another tool to support our menstruating students. We will talk about the importance of rest in the dedicated rest and rejuvenation chapter but most of us are aware that rest is important for our immune system and our hormones. If you are trained in yoga *nidra*, I highly recommend offering it. However, if not, using a guided body scan or creating space for an extended *shavāsana* can be highly beneficial.

There are many variations of poses you can explore and apply these principles to when you teach yoga for menstruating students or clients.

Trying to conceive?

If menstruation has occurred, there is no pregnancy at this time. If your client is trying to conceive this can be a time of grief. Menstruation is not a miscarriage but it can still feel like a loss, and there may be anxiety. Having a period and a menstrual cycle is one of our vital signs of health. The menstrual cycle is our ovulatory cycle and fertility cycle. Honouring the sacredness of the body's natural rhythm and flow may be challenging yet also an empowering perspective during the time of trying to conceive. Allowing the client to grieve is important if that is what they need. Otherwise, you can simply follow the regular menstrual yoga as described above.

For your own and your clients' awareness, remember that there is no evidence that yoga or exercise causes miscarriage. In fact, the National Health Service (2020) recommends keeping up regular exercise, with some precautions, throughout pregnancy. It also confirms that exercise isn't harmful to the baby but can be a support during pregnancy. However, I always recommend yoga teachers to train in pregnancy yoga or to refer to a pregnancy yoga teacher if working with pregnant students as there are significant changes to the body and hormones we need to be aware of.

Yoga during the follicular phase

The follicular phase is the time after menstruation until ovulation. In some medical papers and textbooks, the follicular phase includes menstruation as well. Depending on your students, you can include some of the ideas from this section towards the end of your client's bleeding phase.

When the period begins, we are in a low hormone phase. Both oestrogen and progesterone are at the lowest point, but oestrogen starts to increase during the follicular phase. As a quick reminder, oestrogen can make us feel happier, boosting the feel-good hormones serotonin and dopamine. Your students may feel more adventurous, stronger and energized in their practice.

Oestrogen has anabolic qualities, meaning it helps growth. We can take advantage of these muscle-building qualities when oestrogen is high in the follicular phase and around ovulation. Some studies (Knowles *et al.* 2019) suggest that oestrogen is part of muscle repair and restoration. Another study (Oosthuyse & Bosch 2010) shows improved performance in cycling in the late follicular phase. We might not be cycling in yoga classes but I still found the study interesting regarding the effect on performance.

These findings correspond with *Āyurvedic* wisdom perfectly.

The follicular phase is the *Āyurvedic kapha doṣa* phase. *Kapha doṣa* is very similar to oestrogen. If we think of oestrogen as the female hormone, *kapha doṣa* is what gives the goddess-like qualities of voluptuousness, sensuality and fertility. *Kapha*'s qualities include building up and growth, just like oestrogen's anabolic qualities. People with a majority of *kapha* in their constitution have stamina and endurance. They may gain weight quicker and find it harder to lose weight, but they also appear stronger and more muscular.

These are the positive qualities everybody has in the follicular phase, therefore it's the perfect time to include anything to support muscle growth, strength and maybe to be a bit more adventurous in the practice.

What to avoid during the follicular phase

Nothing! This is the time when *kapha doṣa* gives strength and a more positive mindset. People with plenty of *pitta* in their constitution will highly likely take advantages and potentially push themselves too much. Teaching these type-A personalities, you can encourage the stability aspect of *kapha doṣa.* It is the time to enjoy a stronger practice but remind your students of the necessity of rest and restoration too to create balance.

Vāta people will enjoy new, creative and different aspects of the practice at the follicular phase, as long as you can keep them focused. They may be overly enthusiastic but unlike *pitta* personalities, they can easily get distracted again. This is a very good time for *vāta* people to build up strength and muscle mass. This will also support bone health, which can be an issue later in life, specifically for *vāta*-dominant individuals.

Kapha-dominant people can truly enjoy the follicular phase, but if there is a tendency to laziness, congestion, sluggishness, weight gain, or feeling low, they need encouragement to keep moving. Steady fluid *sūryanamaskāra* (sun salutations) or dynamic flow classes are perfect. And if they are looking to build up strength, add in arm balancing too.

Setting the mood for the yoga class during the follicular phase

Bring an attitude of motivation and encouragement. This is the time for strength, fun, dynamic movement, arm balancing and inversions. Keeping in mind that we are all unique individuals, reflect on the characteristics of the three *doṣas* (see above) to accommodate your students.

Āyurveda doesn't recommend hot yoga or yoga in a heated room because it will aggravate *pitta doṣa* unnecessarily. Yet, this is the phase where we can encourage the warming *ujjâyî prāṇayāma* for *kapha* or *vāta* individuals if appropriate. *Pitta* people generally have enough heat already and can use a softer approach to the breath as a meditative focus.

What we do now will affect the rest of this cycle and the cycles to come. It's about balance. Don't push yourself or your students just because it's the follicular phase. Include rest and relaxation here as well.

Intentions during the follicular time

Energetically and physically this is the time of growth. The moon is growing and the uterine lining is building up. What are we inviting to grow in our lives? Are we ready to receive? How are we preparing our nest or environment for what's to come? This could be the preparation for planting seeds of intentions, projects, inspirations and creations we want to grow. Or perhaps even a pregnancy. *Kapha* is nurturing like Mother Nature. How do we embody the abundance of Mother Nature now and during ovulation?

Let's practise some yoga

Bearing in mind that we all have different needs and constitutions, this is generally when we can embrace a dynamic and physically strong practice. It's time for a mindful yet challenging *vinyāsa* yoga class. Dynamic or *vinyāsa* flow are great to get any stagnant *kapha* moving, plus we have the stamina and endurance with a balanced *kapha*.

As *kapha* is cool and can get sluggish and heavy, we treat, or balance, it with opposites, such as *Sūryanamaskāra* (sun salutations) and *vinyāsa* flows. *Sūryanamaskāra* embraces the warming and solar energy, counteracting any excess cool *kapha*. Include core awareness practices, challenging arm balancing, inversions and extra strength-based classes, as we have the energy and power due to the increasing oestrogen and it being a *kapha*-dominant time.

In the follicular phase, we can encourage circulation and stimulation to the area around the ovaries, encouraging healthy ovulation. This could be through twists, core work and backbends.

Prāṇayāma

Because *kapha* is cool, we can enjoy a slightly warming *ujjâyî prāṇayāma* as a way to focus our attention and intention. It is also a time of strength and power, so more energetic practices such as *bhastrikā* (bellows breath) and *kapālabhāti* (skull-shining breath) are useful. These *prāṇayāmas* are generally good for *kapha* people as they are stimulating, dynamic and move stagnant *kapha*. The seat of *kapha* is the lungs and *prāṇayāmas* are highly recommended for vitiated *kapha*.

If students, such as *pitta* types, tend to push themselves or get overly excited from increased *vāta*, implement balancing *prāṇayāma*. *Brāmari* (bumblebee) breath has a calming effect on the nervous system. Personally, I love *nāḍīśōdhana* (alternate nostril breathing) because it is balancing for all the *doṣas* at any time.

Commencing the yoga class

It's always good to start a class with a bit of grounding and connecting with body and breath, letting go of what we do not need to bring onto the mat. Start either seated or in *shavāsana*, with however you usually commence the class. This may be with chanting, *mantra*, breathing or meditation.

Sequencing

SŪRYANAMASKĀRA (SUN SALUTATIONS)

Have fun sequencing your *vinyāsa* or your standing creative flow. This is a great time to encourage strength through plank poses, *vasiṣṭhāsana* (side plank variations), *chaturaṅgadaṇḍāsana* and staying in your standing poses or core-activating *āsana* for endurance.

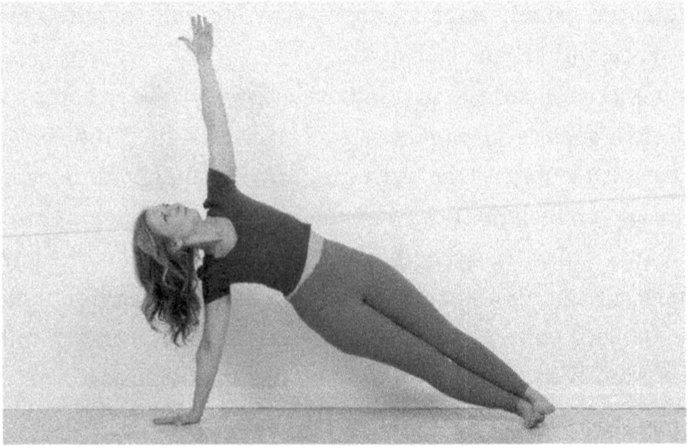

Vasiṣṭhāsana

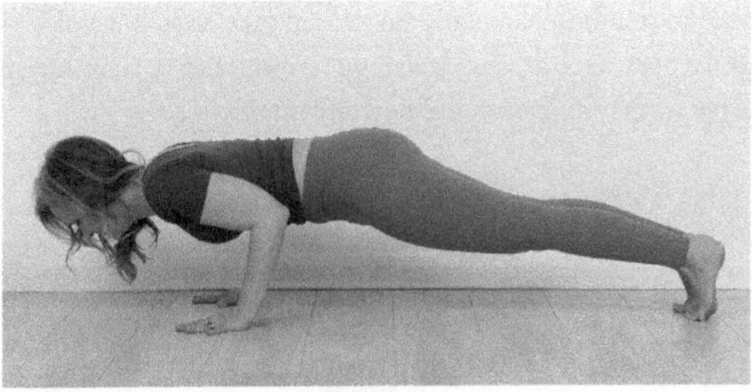

Chaturaṅgadaṇḍāsana

STANDING POSES

Standing poses are excellent to explore alignment, mobility and stability. In the follicular phase, we have the opportunity to increase strength and build muscles. Yoga might not be about physical performance or appearance but many of our students come to class as part of their exercise routine. As a holistic practice, yoga is also about having a healthy body to experience life through.

When warmed up, add in arm strength with yoga push-ups, *chaturaṅga-daṇḍāsana*, and arm balances. Have fun with *adhomukhavṛkṣāsana* (handstand) and *piñchhamayūrāsana* (forearmstand) if you enjoy teaching these.

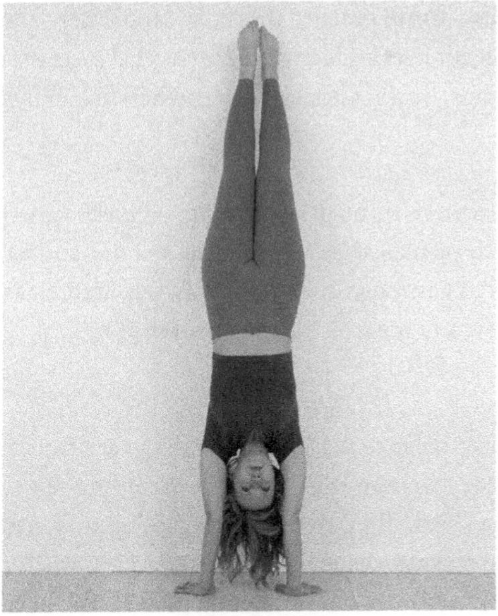

Adhomukhavṛkṣāsana

Bring in some standing balancing poses that take advantage of *kapha*'s stability and support, such as *vīrabhadrāsana* 3 (warrior 3), standing splits, and find creative ways to move up and down from the floor.

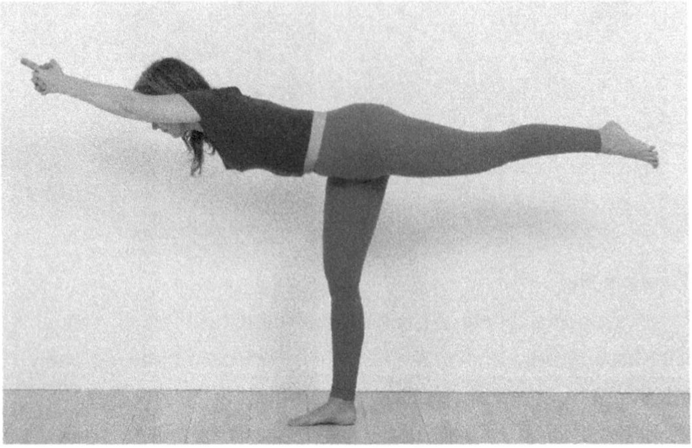

Vīrabhadrāsana 3

This is *kapha* time so we teach with supportive encouragement.

In the follicular phase, you can be as creative as you like. There are no contraindications specifically for this time. And indeed, if anyone wants to enjoy a super easy restful practice that is fine too. There are other elements and influences in our lives aside from the menstrual cycle to take into account such as the seasons, weather, time of day and how the individual is feeling.

CORE FIRE

Activate core awareness through *navāsana* (boat pose) variations, planks and *vasiṣṭhāsana* (side planks). We are increasing stamina and building muscular strength thanks to oestrogen and *kapha doṣa* but what else would your students like to grow and build? It isn't all about the physical.

TWISTING

Seated twists, arm balance twists and standing twists have all the benefits we know of already from regular yoga. They offer mobility of the spine and openness of the chest. They compress the abdominal area and provide a mini-abdominal massage depending on the intention and how it is practised. You can add compression using a rolled-up towel or blanket or the student's fists at the lower abdomen in the area of the ovaries. From an *Āyurvedic* perspective, we are creating a healthy blood supply and circulation to the pelvic organs through the chosen *āsana*.

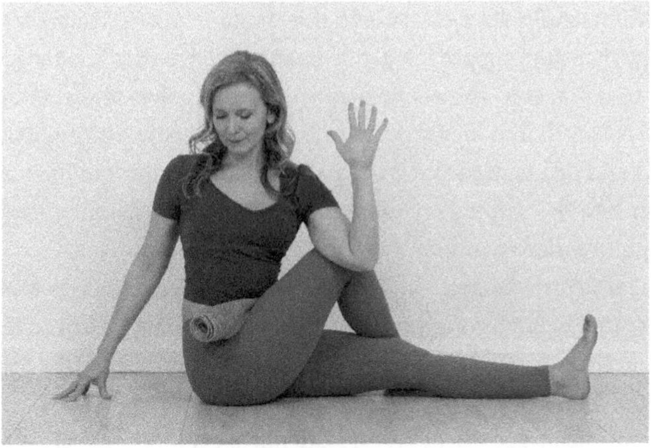

Seated twist with a rolled-up towel at the lower abdomen

BACKBENDING

It's all about balance and we want to open up and create space too. Backbends and lateral (side) stretches are generally recommended for excess *kapha*, as *kapha doṣa* is associated with the lungs. This is also why breathing practices are highly recommended for *kapha* types.

This is another opportunity to open the front of the pelvis, the hip flexors and the abdominal area. This might also be the time to offer options of deeper backbend variations such as *dhanurāsana* (full wheel).

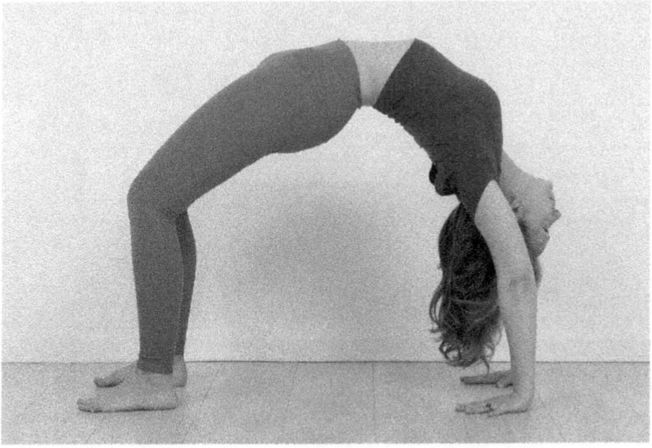

Dhanurāsana

OPEN HEART = OPEN HIPS

With all the standing and potentially stronger practices the body has naturally activated the pelvic floor and abdominal engagement. This is something our body automatically does on its own but in some poses, teachers will also encourage that extra support. A gentle *mūlabandha*, pelvic floor engagement, is a way to connect to the pelvic diaphragm and pelvis to create the blood flow and strength that are important for pelvic health. This will also affect the fascia and ligaments around the pelvis, which connect to the uterus and ovaries and to the respiratory diaphragm. Our pelvic diaphragm relates to the respiratory diaphragm.

It is also essential to relax and release any tension here. Tight muscles are restrictive and do not have optimal blood flow or mobility. We need to learn to relax the pelvic area. Relaxing the pelvic diaphragm may affect the respiratory diaphragm and help us breathe more fully with more ease.

I always encourage teachers and students to explore pelvic floor practices understanding when to relax and when to engage. A pose like *kapotāsana* (pigeon pose) is a good pose for this, as is *malāsana* (yogīc squat). In both these poses you can teach to engage the pelvic floor and at the same time feel the head of the femurs (thigh bones) hug into the acetabulum (hip sockets) and then allowing the body and pelvic diaphragm to relax. It's an exaggerated movement in which we can ask our students to find where they need the stability of engagement or the softness of release.

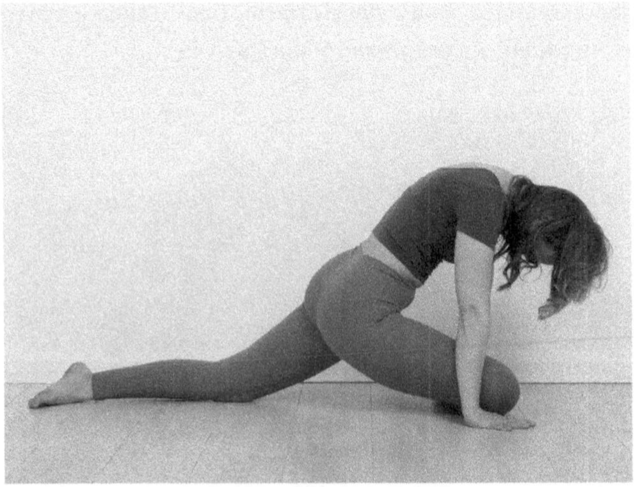

Draw the thighbones into the hip sockets and engage the pelvic floor to rise

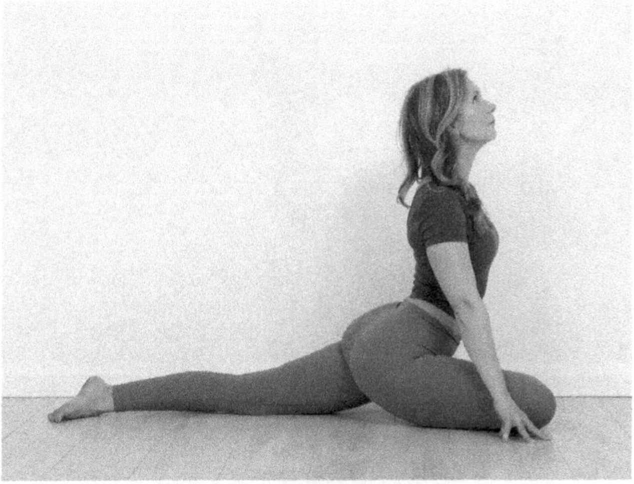

Release and soften to lower down

Where we use lots of props and softness in the menstrual phase we can work with muscular support and strength as we move into hip openers such as *kapotāsana* (pigeon pose), lunges or lizard poses during the follicular phase.

COOLING DOWN

At the end of this more solar energy class, we create balance with lunar sequencing. It's all about balance. Add in hip-opening poses, seated forward bends, restorative twists and any inversions you usually offer, such as *śīrṣāsana* (headstand) and *sālambasarvāṅgāsana* (shoulderstand).

We can also offer more advanced breathing practices and meditations with *kumbhaka* (breath retention) and *bandhas* (seals or locks).

Relaxation is restorative and rejuvenating. Regardless of where we are in the menstrual cycle, most of us need to restore and rest. This can be a challenge for many but relaxation is powerful and will support our hormonal and *doṣic* balance. Resting during the follicular phase will affect the menstrual and premenstrual phases too, which we explore in depth in Chapter 13 on rest and rejuvenation.

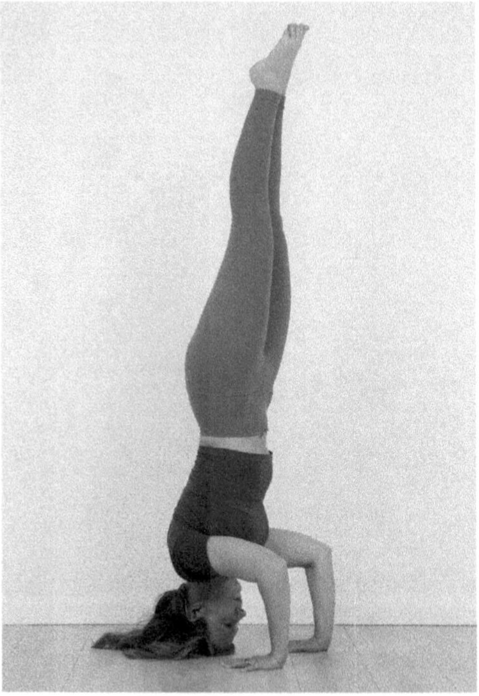

Tripod variation of śīrṣāsana

Trying to conceive?

If you teach someone trying to conceive, remember that the sperm can live inside the reproductive tract for up to around five days. Although ovulation happens on just one day, the sperm can happily live until ovulation day and then potentially fertilize the egg.

Although there is no evidence that any form of exercise including yoga can negatively affect the sperm or the potential fertilization, you can suggest a softer and gentler practice at this time and until the person knows if they are pregnant or not.

If we want to conceive we can encourage the endometrium to build up. In *Āyurveda*, this means honouring *kapha doṣa* and specifically building up *ojas*. We looked briefly at the concept of *ojas* in the introduction to *Āyurveda*. *Ojas* is nourishing, building, juiciness and is our immunity. It is lustre and glow. It is cooling and sweet like the luminosity of the full moon, like ghee or honey.

In this case, it is important not to burn out the *ojas*. We need to keep it nice and cool. This relates to our yoga practice as well as general lifestyle, stress and diet. Although there is strength and stamina at this time if someone is trying to conceive, leave out some of the very solar and heating practices.

Yoga during the ovulation time

Ovulation is the day when an egg is released from a follicle from either of the ovaries into the uterine tube. Oestrogen peaks just before ovulation. This triggers a surge of luteinizing hormone and then the egg is released. The process takes about 24 hours. We can say ovulation is a result of the peaks of oestrogen, follicle-stimulating hormone and luteinizing hormone.

Ovulation happens around the middle of the menstrual cycle. In a textbook 28-day cycle, this would be day 14, but people have longer or shorter cycles. It is also worth considering that the luteal phase is usually always the same length but the follicular phase can change in the individual.

Although this is a short phase, the build-up is steady. Our students might enjoy this ovulatory energy a few days before and after the actual ovulation.

At the time around ovulation hormone levels are high and most people feel really good. There is a natural sense of confidence and energy. It's the time for a potential pregnancy, and oestrogen along with *kapha doṣa* energy may make us feel extra juicy, sexy and sensual too.

It is the time of the month when we have the most testosterone in our circulation. Testosterone is generally thought of as a male sex hormone but it is also part of female physiology and health. It increases the feel-good hormone dopamine and is part of healthy libido, orgasms and sexual wellbeing. It contributes to muscular and bone health.

In *Āyurveda*, *kapha doṣa* has been building up. Here we can connect *kapha* to the qualities of love, sensuality and fertility. *Kapha* is the element of earth and water. It is juiciness and flow. There is stamina and endurance. *Kapha* is cool in temperature.

There are suggestions that certain hormonal changes contribute to more flexibility in our ligaments around ovulation. This makes sense from an *Āyurvedic* perspective. Although *kapha* is stable and structured, it is also the soft watery fluid element. The stretchiness and flexibility could be partly due to *kapha* and the *kapha*-like hormones of rising oestrogen. From a Western perspective, research is scanty, contradictory and of variable quality. Some studies suggest that female athletes are more likely to injure their anterior crucial ligament just before and at ovulation. In contrast, other papers suggest that injury is more likely in the premenstrual and menstrual phases (Melegario *et al.* 2006; Herzberg *et al.* 2017; Martin *et al.* 2021; Beynnon & Shultz 2008; Wojtys *et al.* 1998).

Another study (Miyazaki & Maeda 2022) investigating changes in hamstring flexibility found that the 'range of motion and passive torque at the onset of pain were significantly increased during the ovulatory and luteal phases compared with the follicular phase'. It seems the increased 'flexibility during the ovulatory and luteal phases' is 'influenced by fluctuations in sex hormones'. The jury is still out on these issues although we can consider the watery fluid element of *kapha doṣa* when we teach our yoga classes. More importantly, we can let our students observe any shifts they may have through the cycle and instruct accordingly. If there is a sense of looseness, hypermobility or instability, we focus on stability and support to avoid injuries.

Ovulation is a shift and movement of the mature follicle releasing an egg. Any movement and mobility are governed by *vāta*. *Vāta* is part of the ovulation process releasing the egg from the follicle in the ovary to the uterine tube.

Vāta is associated with pain. As the *Āyurvedic* saying goes: where there is pain there is *vāta*. Some people experience pain or a twinge at either one of their ovaries during ovulation. In Germany, this dull ache or cramp is called *mittelschmerz*, translated as middle (of the cycle) pain. It usually lasts a few hours but can be a couple of days.

What to avoid during the ovulatory phase

In a way, the ovulation phase is a continuation of the follicular phase. Or perhaps the pinnacle. There isn't anything you need to avoid in the yoga practice. This will be about the individual's intentions and energy, just like in the follicular phase.

Intentions during the ovulatory time

If we relate ovulation to the moon cycle, it would be the full moon. The full moon is abundant, lustrous, bright and full. It is the peak of the moon cycle, and often thought of as a time of manifestation. During the waxing moon phase, things or intentions grow; at the full moon, it all comes to fruition.

It is the same with the inner moon cycle. It is the time of manifestation. We may or may not want to manifest a pregnancy. Either way, the ovulatory and full moon energy can be a time of creation and abundance.

The full moon also shines brightly in the darkness of the night. Sometimes this is also a challenging time. What is hiding in the shadows? What has been allowed to grow in the darkness of our mind or our ego? What have we been trying to shy away from or hide under the carpet, in the darkness? The illuminating full-moon glow may shine its light on those shadows – and so may our abundant ovulation energy. It is an excellent opportunity to befriend our shadows.

Let's practise some yoga

Here we can go two ways. We can continue with the power, strength and stamina of the follicular phase. It's a time of confidence and creativity, so any stronger practice can work well to direct and focus the increased *kapha doṣa*, oestrogen and testosterone. Maybe the peak pose or focus that's been worked through the follicular phase gets to shine abundantly here at ovulation.

Alternatively, we can embrace the sensual, soft and fluid feminine energy of fertility, oestrogen and *kapha* as the earth Goddess. This can be a softer, circular or spiralling flow – the opposite of the often taught, linear, alignment-based yoga classes. Allow for the students' own intuitive movements; think more somatic movement rather than a strongly structured sequencing.

Start rocking the pelvis and making other pelvic movements to bring energy and awareness to this often neglected area. We are sedentary humans and many of us have tightness in our hip flexors and pelvis in general. We often slouch, which contributes to a tight and constricted pelvic floor. With anxiety or stress thrown in, we tighten our pelvic floor and abdomen even further. This affects our breathing, digestion and pelvic health including our pelvic organs and therefore the menstrual cycle. Remember, everything is connected. The muscles around our pelvis and the fascia that supports the uterus and ovaries are connected. Freeing the pelvis with pelvic tilts, rocking and swaying might also support our pelvic organs and therefore our cycle, as well as our general wellbeing.

If you play music, introduce soft beats and sensual rhythm.

Āsana and sequencing

If you or your ovulating students prefer to focus and direct their *pitta* fire with a strong dynamic class, continue with the follicular phase sequencing ideas. They may have the confidence to be a bit more adventurous and try new things or a different or more advanced (for them) variation of a yoga pose or sequence.

Because life, in general, can be very linear and masculine (in energy), I like to introduce some more fluid, feminine circular energy. This is often what we teach in pregnancy yoga classes – more spiralling flow and allowing the body to move as it wishes. This may not be for everybody and it is not textbook yoga, but it does connect with the qualities of ovulation, the full moon, and oestrogen peaking for the potential for pregnancy and *kapha* sensuality.

Prāṇayāma

The *prāṇayāma* practice could be the dynamic *kapālabhāti* (skull-shining breath) or *bhastrikā* (bellows breath) as suggested in the follicular phase to energize *kapha*, but also to strengthen and connect with the core. If you enjoy a more soothing practice, I suggest a gentle *ujjâyî prāṇayāma* or the balancing *nāḍīśōdhana* (alternate nostril breathing).

Commencing the class

Instead of sitting rigidly in meditation as you start the class, allow for gently swaying, rocking or circulating. It is not a directed alignment cue, but rather inviting our students to let their bodies move. It's also a good time to introduce the awareness of the pelvic floor and moving from the pelvis, for example moving from one sitting bone towards the pubic bone to the other sitting bone and the tailbone. Continue this circular movement in both directions. This is moving from the pelvis rather than directing the rotation of the head of the femur in the hip socket. Through this movement, you connect with the pelvis and the pelvic floor.

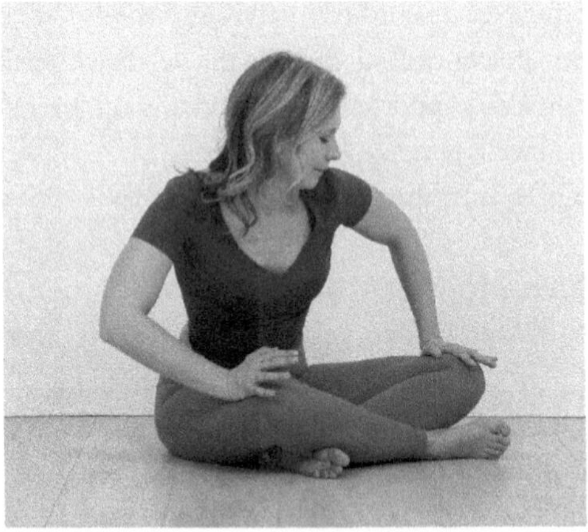

Enjoy circular and fluid movements with no rigid rules or alignment cues

Hands can rest in *yoni* or *shakti mudrā* near the lower abdomen over the womb space or on the knees. I also like one hand on womb space and the other hand on heart space (anatomically the sternum not the actual heart).

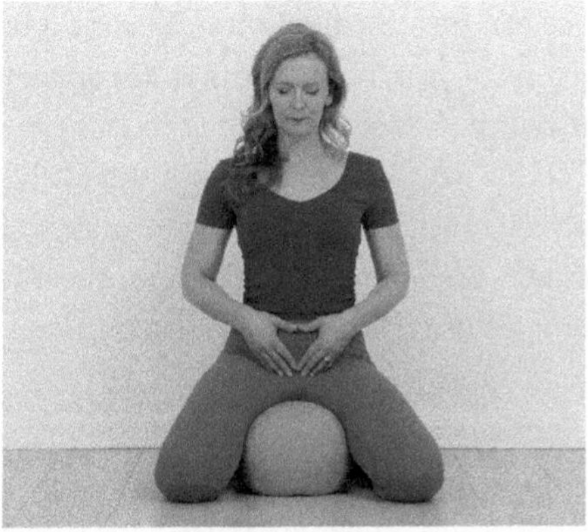

Yoni mudrā creates a triangle shape with the index fingers pointing down, thumbs together and hands on the lower abdomen

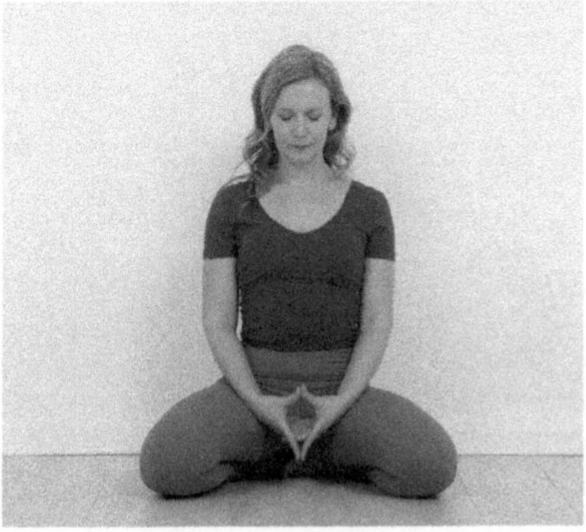

Shakti mudrā: interlace the finger. Index fingers extend and point down. Tip of the thumbs touch pointing up

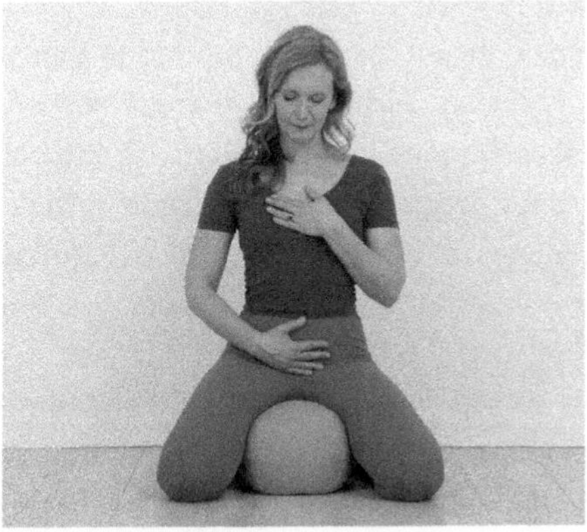

Gently rest one hand over the centre of the chest and the other over the womb space

This seated practice can be a meditation or become a breathing practice. Depending on the time of year, if the studio is hot or cool, and on the individual, you can introduce *sheetali prāṇayāma* (cooling breath). The cooling nurturing energy connects us to our *ojas* and the quality of 'building up'. It's the cooling glow and nectar of the full moon, ghee (clarified butter) and honey. It is the refined *kapha doṣa* and the fullness of the endometrium. *Nāḍīśōdhana* (alternate nostril breathing) is also excellent to create balance.

Sequencing

FLUID MOVEMENTS

Hands-and-knees poses and lunges are perfect for students to explore the spontaneous non-aligned flow in their bodies. Rocking forwards and backwards, making circles or figures of eight are brilliant ways to embrace a sensual natural somatic flow.

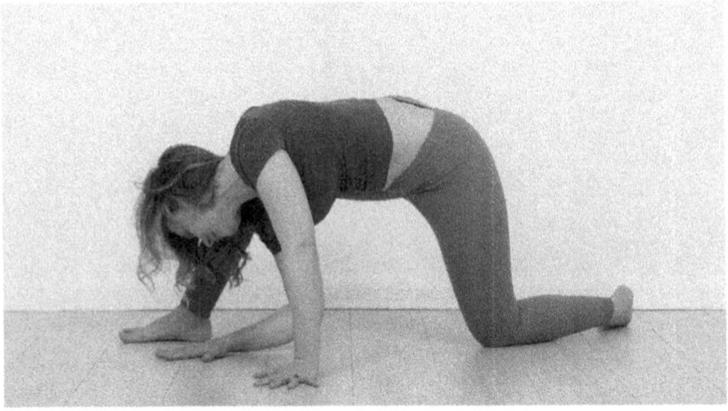

In a lunge position, allow the body to flow in circular movements

SALUTATIONS

If ovulation happens to be on the actual full moon then *chandranāmaskar* (moon salutation) is perfect. Although *chandranāmaskar* may warm up the body, the energy is to honour and connect with the cooling, nourishing lunar energy. So even if we are at any other time in the outer moon cycle, *chandranāmaskar* is a good way to start a more structured or familiar flow.

STANDING POSES

There are no rules! You might just keep it fluid and almost dance-like. Or perhaps more of a meditative flow. Let it be playful. Dancing warriors where you flow from extended side angle pose to reverse warrior is a great addition to bring playfulness and flow into the yoga class.

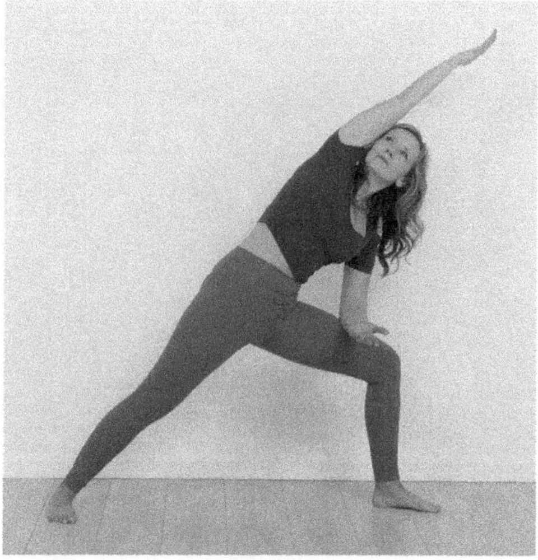

Extended side angle pose with either hand on the floor or block, or forearm on the thigh

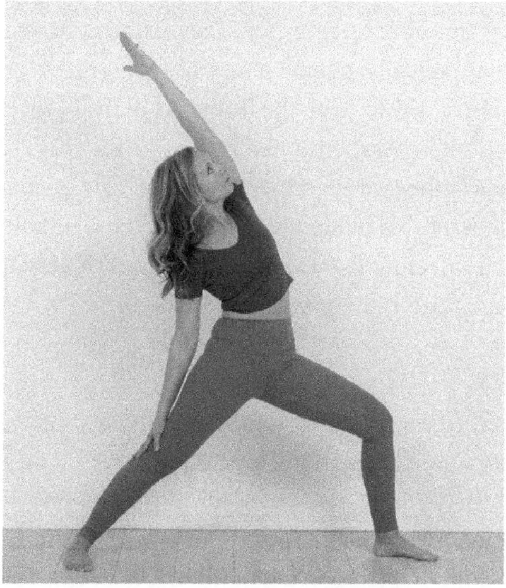

Keeping the front knee bend flow into reverse warrior pose

Goddess squat, or horse stand, is powerful and strong. It is fierce and feminine. You can offer a pulsation of straightening the legs and bending the knees again. Add in pelvic floor engagement as you rise, and release as the knees bend for more pelvic awareness.

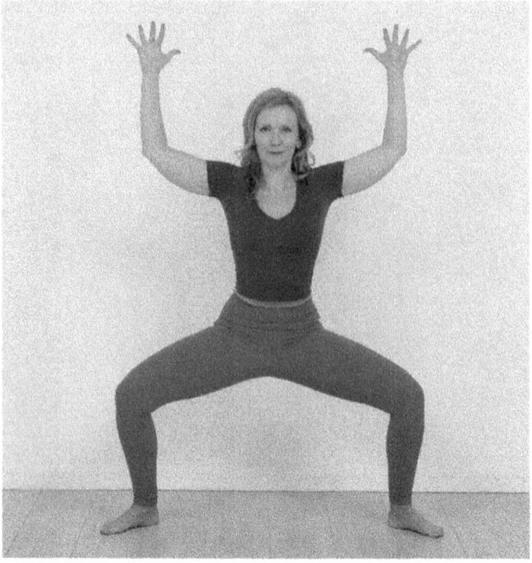

Goddess squat can be practised with different arm variations

BACKBENDING

A backbend can symbolize opening up to opportunity, to receive and potentially conceive symbolically, maybe a new idea, a creative project or a baby. Backbending is also a way to open the front gate of the body, of the hip flexors and the lower abdomen. As mentioned earlier, we are very sedentary and our hips get tight. So whether we open them in a lunge, hip opener or a backbend, we start to counteract this tendency. This could be a standing *natarajāsana* (dancer's pose) or kneeling *ustrāsana* (camel pose) or perhaps *dhanurāsana* (full wheel). There is no right or wrong pose here.

FORWARD BENDS

Forward bending, either seated or standing, provides some gentle compression on the abdomen. Although the uterus and ovaries are situated lower at the pelvic bowl, they might also get some compression in forward bends. Around ovulation time, we can add additional stimulation by placing a double fist just above the pubic bone when folding forward. This is particularly effective in *bālāsana* (child's pose) and could be applied in twists as well, with part of a small rolled-up blanket. I wouldn't suggest this if your student is trying to conceive though. If that's the case, create lots of space instead.

You can continue the fluid and more sensuous movement in *upaviṣṭakoṇāsana* (wide-angle seated forward bend), making circular or rocking movements from the pelvis. Introduce cat-cow-like movement from the pelvis in lunges and *kapotāsana* (pigeon pose variations) too.

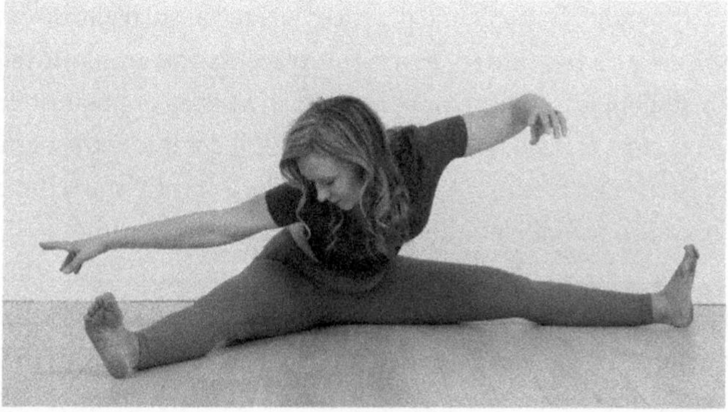

Upaviṣṭakoṇāsana variation with circular flow from the pelvis through the arms

By flexing and extending the lower abdomen and pelvic area we connect with the muscles, fascia and pelvic organs. This is the area of *apāna vāyu*. We always want *apāna vāyu* to be balanced. *Apāna vāyu* may be associated with menstruation but if there is an obstruction it will also affect ovulation. The action or mobilization of the release of the egg is partly due to *vāta doṣa*, as movement is a *vāta* quality.

Even if there is no interest in procreation or wanting to conceive, ovulation is an important event for fertility, our wellbeing and our cycle. Practising *āsana* to balance *apāna vāyu* is a way to support all functions of the reproductive system and the *yoni*.

RELAXATION

Shavāsana is sometimes said to be the most challenging *āsana* as we are doing nothing. There is nothing to focus or concentrate on. We are *being*, not *doing*. Perhaps initiate enquiry or meditations to connect with the full moon energy of nourishment, sweetness and abundance, regardless of the actual lunar phase. This restores and rejuvenates.

Trying to conceive?

Ovulation is the only time a person can conceive. Sperm can live in the reproductive tract for a few days beforehand and then fertilization will happen on the day of ovulation. If your student is on a fertility journey, this is the perfect time to enjoy more sensuous fluid movements to encourage the watery fluid element and the building energy of *kapha doṣa*.

Although there is no evidence that any form of movement practice can affect the fertilization process, it makes sense from an *Āyurvedic* perspective to enhance and encourage *ojas*-building qualities and healthy *kapha doṣa*. You do not want any potentially depleting practices when you are trying to encourage pregnancy, create a new life (or several), a placenta and amniotic fluid.

If your student is feeling anxious or is on an assisted or medicated fertility journey they may choose not to practise at all. If so, this is the perfect time to enjoy rest and relaxation. A person who has recently started their yoga journey may also feel more vulnerable or insecure at this time.

Pregnancy is not an illness or a disease. It is a time of incredible hormonal, physical as well as *doṣic* changes taking place; therefore, I would always suggest that a pregnant student is guided by a yoga teacher qualified in teaching prenatal yoga.

Yoga during the luteal phase

The luteal phase begins after ovulation. Some people sense a definite shift post-ovulation, although for most people, the phases flow into each other more subtly. The actual luteal phase lasts around 12–14 days but can be longer or shorter.

Several things happen during this part of the menstrual cycle. In the follicular phase, a follicle matures and finally ruptures to release an egg at ovulation. The follicle left becomes what is called the corpus luteum and is a transient endocrine organ. This increases the production of the hormone progesterone, which affects the luteal phase. The corpus luteum will start to shrink and dissolve 9–11 days after ovulation, unless pregnancy occurs.

One reason that progesterone builds up the endometrium is to prepare for a potential pregnancy. It relaxes the uterus to prohibit contractions, which could reject a fertilized egg. Progesterone can be a relaxant of smooth muscles in general, such as the intestines, where it can influence our digestion and potentially lead to constipation. Progesterone helps to build up the endometrium in case there is a fertilized egg to be received and embedded into the uterine lining. This hormone also has slightly heating properties. The basal temperature during the luteal phase is higher than at any other time.

Oestrogen remains high in the early luteal phase. This helps to build up and create a structure just like *kapha doṣa*.

Both progesterone and oestrogen contribute to the thickening of the endometrial lining, which is important for pregnancy. But after 9–11 days, progesterone and oestrogen decline, preparing us for a new cycle and a new opportunity to release the endometrial lining with the menstruation phase. The sudden drop of hormones can cause fatigue, strong emotional experiences and more intense premenstrual syndromes.

Another hormone rising in the luteal phase is relaxin, generally recognized as a pregnancy hormone released from the placenta. It is commonly believed to relax the ligaments in pregnancy so that the body can expand to support the growing uterus. It has also, until recently, been thought to be the reason that pelvic pain, and ligament pain in general, is common in pregnancy. Now, research suggests this may not be the case (Petersen, Hvidman & Uldbjerg 1994; Hansen *et al.* 1996) and that the pain could be the result of other hormonal and anatomical changes. I also want to point out that we all have relaxin. In male physiology, it is found in the prostate gland rather than primarily secreted from the corpus luteum of the ovaries in female physiology (Agoulnik 2007). The role of relaxin includes bone remodelling and healing of injured ligaments and skeletal muscles. Some (limited) research indicates that relaxin is associated with posterior pelvic and lumbar pain (Wreje *et al.* 1995). We may have students who observe they feel more flexible in the luteal phase perhaps due to increased relaxin levels.

In *Āyurveda*, we can compare this part of the cycle to *pitta doṣa*. *Pitta* is fire, heat and transformation. Pitta is action – creating opportunity for conception or opportunity for a new cycle with another menstrual phase. *Pitta* is also about being sharp and focused. It is the light so we can see clearly. Excess *pitta* is overheating, which can manifest as perspiration and increased body temperature, hot flushes and inflammation, but also as hot temper, irritability, anger and frustration. Many premenstrual syndromes could be caused by excess or imbalanced *pitta doṣa*.

There are several studies on yoga for PMS, with one study (Wu *et al.* 2015) suggesting 'that women with PMS could attend short-term yoga exercise in the luteal phase to make themselves feel better and maintain a better attention level'.

What to avoid during the luteal phase

In our yoga practice, we can embrace the positive of *pitta* but be careful not to overheat and increase it. As progesterone and *pitta* can increase body temperature, it is best to avoid hot yoga.

Remember that everybody is different. A *pitta*-dominant person may feel a lot hotter and more irritated than a chilled out, cool and calm *kapha* personality. There is also a difference between the earlier luteal phase where oestrogen and progesterone are still high and just before the menstrual phase where the hormones drop.

In the discussion about ovulation, I shared some research on anterior crucial ligament (ACL) injury and the potential connection to the menstrual cycle. Some research suggests that injuries are more common around ovulation. Other research indicates it is more common in the premenstrual phase. This is why menstrual cycle awareness and tracking is so helpful. How does the individual experience these hormonal and *doṣic* shifts? If they know they feel more 'loose' or hypermobile when premenstrual then we can make sure we focus on alignment and support at that specific time.

There is some evidence suggesting that coordination can be more challenging during the luteal phase too (Bayer & Hausmann 2012; Fridén, *et al.* 2006). My personal experience is that I tend to mix up my rights and lefts when teaching yoga classes during my late luteal phase. I confuse both myself and my students! But it's a sign for me that my period is due soon, and I know I can use my *pitta* sharpness, and focus my mind on getting it right.

This is also the time when I feel less stable and structured in my body. I like deep stretching, especially in my hips and hamstrings during this time. It feels as if I am more flexible. This corresponds with the research on how we may be more flexible, and prone to injury, during the luteal phase. One such study (Myklebust *et al.* 1998) revealed that the Norwegian handball team experienced more ACL injuries in the luteal phase. However, this study contradicts other studies indicating that ACL injuries are more common just before and at the ovulatory phase.

In conclusion, avoid heating practices, don't overstretch, and be aware that the capacity for high-intensity, strength-building and endurance exercise may be lower than during the follicular phase. With the clarity and sharpness of *pitta doṣa*, we can embrace detailed alignment, structure and focus through the yoga practices.

Setting the mood for the yoga class during the luteal phase

We can relate this phase to the waning moon. This is especially helpful for those not menstruating. Just after the full moon, the glow and abundance are still visible, and the hormones are still high. But when the moon starts to become less and less visible, so too are the hormones. Where in the actual lunar or moon cycle are you right now? What are you ready to implement or impregnate into your life (early phase)? And what are you ready to release (late phase)? Are you ready to dive into the darkness and be in the reflective phase of your shadows?

Let's practise some yoga

At the beginning of the luteal phase, we still have high hormones and more energy. Here we can enjoy the *pitta* sharpness and fire along with the strength and stamina of *kapha*. This is while there is still increased testosterone, oestrogen and progesterone around. We want to be mindful not to increase *pitta doṣa*. Excess *pitta* is heat and inflammation. This can lead to feeling physically hot, including hot flushes. But it can also mean heat as anger and irritability, which are some of the common premenstrual symptoms.

Then the hormones drop. The basal temperature in our body increases and we get hot and bothered. It's time to slow down and calm our practice so as not to aggravate *pitta doṣa*.

Unless your student is trying to conceive, this is an excellent time to focus on 'letting go'. We are preparing for the shedding of the uterine lining at menstruation and *raktamokṣa*, or the blood cleansing process, from an *Āyurvedic* perspective. With that in mind, we can still slow and cool down yet also create some stimulation and circulation at the pelvis. This could include twisting and *bālāsana* (child's pose) variations.

For anyone with water retention, we need to keep moving to support the lymphatic flow. This can include the classic *pawanmuktāsana* sequence from the Bihar School of yoga tradition – circling, flexing and extending the ankles, knees and wrists.

It also includes the wind-releasing exercise. Here, lie supine, inhaling to hug the right knee to the chest, lifting the chest while holding the breath, then releasing with the exhale. Then inhale to hug the left knee and lift the chest, exhale to release, and finally with both knees repeat for a few rounds. This variation is also recommended for anyone with wind. The wind refers to *vāta doṣa* which causes wind (*vāyu*) in the intestines as well as excess *vāta* in the joints, making them achy.

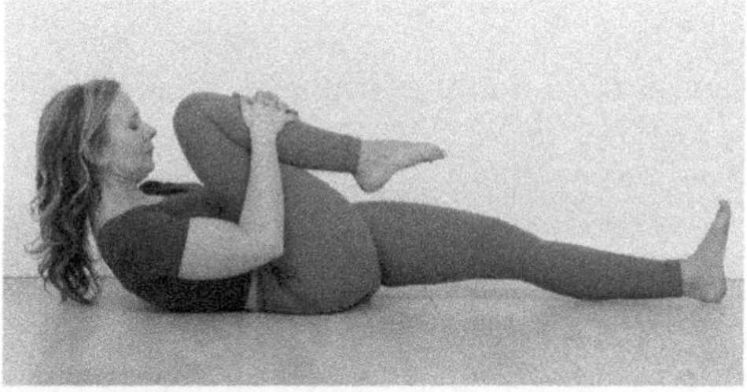

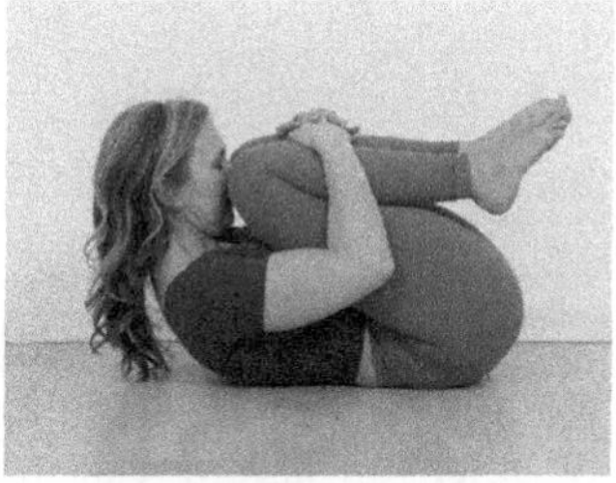

Lie on the back with legs straight (alternatively with knees bend pointing up and feet flat on the floor). Inhale and bend the right knee to the chest. Lift the chest and head. Exhale release. Repeat with the left leg. Repeat by hugging both knees to the chest

Personally, I love the pelvic rocking and circling just before my period. I often get achy around the sacrum, hips and legs in the late luteal phase, and gentle rocking seems to be a way to create mobility, fluidity and flow. On an energetic level, this moving meditation is a way to welcome the next phase of my cycle, to create space and allow menstruation to arrive.

If you use music you can slow it down, with slow beats to focus on alignment and a slower flow.

Āsana and sequencing

We will focus on the early to the mid-luteal phase. In the days before menstruation starts, refer to the menstrual yoga section of slowing down and enjoying a more meditative yoga practice.

Prāṇayāma

At this time, there can be many intense emotions. Breath awareness is a powerful way to calm down, balance and regulate the nervous system. Simple instructions to notice and observe the breath are helpful. Learning diaphragmatic breathing or complete breaths is essential for our emotional and physical wellness. A yoga class is a perfect place to introduce and implement awareness and mindfulness of the breath and how it connects to body and mind.

Aim to balance the heat and the cold. The solar and the lunar. I always like to introduce *nāḍīśōdhana* (alternate nostril breathing). It is perfect whether your students are hot-headed, erratic, anxious or low.

For anger and irritability, *brāmari prāṇayāma* (bumblebee breath) is an excellent way to calm the heated and overactive mind. This is the bumblebee breathing where you hum on the exhale. Humming has been shown to increase parasympathetic tone, meaning it's easier to relax after stress (Ghati *et al.* 2021).

In the later luteal phase, when physical manifestations of discomfort in the pelvis can occur, gentle rocking with *ujjâyî prāṇayāma* can be another way of managing pain.

Commencing the yoga class

Whether you start in relaxation pose, *shavāsana*, or seated meditation, you can begin with focus. *Pitta* finds it easy to focus. I like to introduce a *Kali mudrā* movement meditation and re-introduce the *mudrā* and arm variation through the sequence, for example in *vīrabhadrāsana* 1 (warrior 1) pose. For this variation, which I learned from Shiva Rea, you interlace the fingers, with index fingers pointing up. Inhale to extend the *mudrā* above the head, with the index fingers pointing up. Then 'cut' through as you reach the arms in front of you to heart level. Continue this circular movement with the intention of clearing the path, letting go and seeing clearly. This phase of the cycle is a good time to see through the illusions.

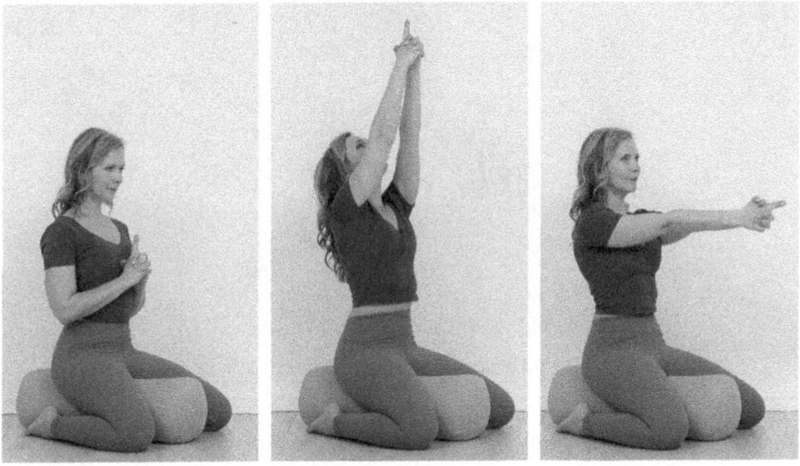

Kali mudrā movement meditation

Sequencing

STARTING THE FLOW

When practising *sūrya* or *chandranamaskāra* (sun or moon salutation) or any other warming up flow or *vinyāsa*, focus on detail and alignment rather than pushing through. In the luteal and ovulatory phases, we think of strengthening and building muscle. Now we need more recovery time. So take time to embrace the basics and foundations of the practice.

STANDING POSES

We can apply *dristhi*, or visual focus, and breath awareness. This is a good way to direct any increased *pitta doṣa*. Again, focus on alignment. *Vīrabhadrāsana* (warrior poses), *utthitapārśvakoṇāsana* (extended side angle), *trikoṇāsana* (triangle pose) and similar poses are excellent to teach physical awareness, detail and the connection of body, breath and mind.

I like using the moving *Kali mudrā* meditation from the beginning of the class in *Vīrabhadrāsana* 1 (warrior 1). This symbolizes warrior goddess Kali clearing the path, demolishing the demons yet being grounded and a protector.

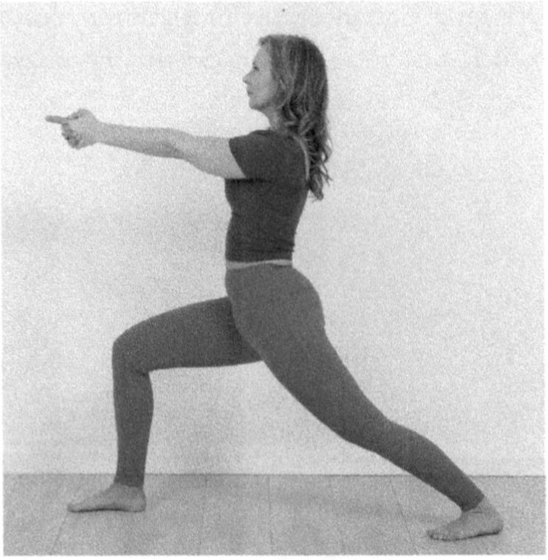

Vīrabhadrāsana 1 with Kali mudrā

Balancing poses can be more challenging in the luteal phase. Yet, we can be in a balancing pose learning to be wobbly and playful and not taking things too seriously. We find our centre, even if everything around us, as well as our hormones, make us feel unstable.

BACKBENDING

The seat of *pitta*, or *agni*, is in the organ of the stomach, including our digestion and digestive juices. It also has a connection with the fire of our core and via the fire element, it associates with the *maṇipūra cakra* or navel centre.

In a way, backbending can open and release some of the constriction and tightness we may feel in our abdomen due to the anger, heat and irritability of *pitta*. Several studies on yoga and menstrual symptoms include and highlight backbends practised as general weekly yoga classes over several months. One study (Rakhshaee 2011) indicated that including cat pose, *matsyāsana* (fish pose) and *bhujaṅgāsana* (cobra pose) in yoga could reduce the severity and the length of painful periods when done in the luteal phase.

FORWARD BENDS

Forward bends are calming and cooling for *pitta doṣa*. In *bālāsana* (child's pose) or any seated forward bend, the practitioner can make a fist with their hands, place it just above the pubic bone and fold over the fist. This creates some compression on the lower belly near the uterus. Breathing deep into this compression is like an abdominal massage. The womb is in the pelvis, which is the seat of *vāta doṣa* and specifically *apāna vāyu*. *Vāta* is dry, cold and light. Bringing warmth, pressure and circulation can support and balance *vāta doṣa* as it prepares for menstruation. The lower abdomen is also where we find our intestines. Intestines and bowel movements are associated with *vāta* – and *apāna vāyu* (remember the downward-moving energy-releasing waste!). Poses such as forward bends help to release excess *vāta* and create balance again.

TWISTING

Although twisting has many benefits I love to include it for menstrual health for the same reasons as forward bends. It offers compression of the lower abdomen and releases excess *vāta*. Perhaps this is one of the reasons yoga is helpful for menstrual symptoms.

ARM BALANCING AND INVERSIONS

At the beginning of the luteal phase, there is still plenty of oestrogen and testosterone giving the endurance and muscular strength for playing around with arm balances and inversions. In the mid to later part of the luteal phase, the playfulness may be replaced with alignment and technique, yet still enjoying and having fun with more challenging poses. There is a point where the energy drops and fatigue sets in. Then, as always, listen to the body and enjoy periods of rest and rejuvenation.

Sālambasarvāṅgāsana (shoulderstand) and *viparīta karaṇī* (legs-up-the-wall) are beautiful, cooling and calming practices often suggested for pelvic health and specifically for the female physiology. Open any yoga book and there are claims of the many benefits specifically for menstrual or female health. Both Iyengar's *Light on Yoga* and Swami Satyananda Saraswati's *Āsana Prāṇayāma Mudrā Bandha* books suggest *sālambasarvāṅgāsana* (shoulderstand) for 'uterine displacement, menstrual trouble' and 'menopause, menstrual disorders and leucorrhoea'. Although *sālambasarvāṅgāsana* (shoulderstand) is an inversion, and I wouldn't suggest it during the menstrual phase as it works against *apāna vāyu*, it is commonly recommended for pelvic health in the yoga community at any other time. We can consider it as a calming yoga pose for the body, mind and hormones. Inversions take the pressure from the internal organs off the pelvic floor and its ligaments, perhaps giving the uterus space to rest, realign or rebalance too. We can enjoy *sālambasarvāṅgāsana* (shoulderstand), if appropriate, at any time except during menses from an *Āyurvedic* and yogīc perspective.

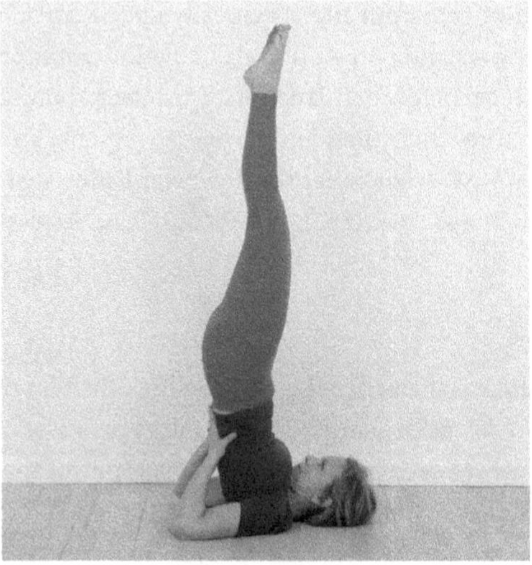

Sālambasarvāṅgāsana

Rest and relaxation

As always, it is so important to rest, rejuvenate and relax and I will go into more detail on this in the next chapter. In the very early luteal phase, we have the strong energy of ovulation and then we drop into the low hormone phase of the premenstrual time and its potential for fatigue and tiredness. When we are tired and exhausted, we need to rest, and we need to rest and restore through the cycle so it doesn't accumulate as a premenstrual syndrome or complete depletion during the menstrual phase.

Pitta is high at this time and needs to rest and cool down. Increased body temperature is one thing but the heat and inflammation of our emotions manifesting as irritability and anger is also an imbalanced pitta symptom. Finding ways for us to restore, build up and rejuvenate helps to potentially reduce PMS as well as prevent discomfort during menstruation.

Vāta doṣa is also active as we move towards menstruation. *Vāta* is movement that can give rise to anxiety and insomnia. *Vāta* is light and needs the stillness and rejuvenating qualities of rest and relaxation – which are the opposite of excess *vāta* qualities.

Excess *kapha doṣa* can manifest as feeling dull and depressed. Water retention, including swollen and painful breasts, is a common *kapha* symptom. Although movement is recommended for *kapha*, we all need rest. For *kapha*, learning to breathe deeply and completely with the diaphragm is useful. In fact, most *prāṇayāma* are excellent for *kapha* as the seat of this *doṣa* is the lungs.

Trying to conceive?

Those trying to conceive may feel anxious to know if fertilization has happened. This is a time of waiting. If someone is on an assisted fertility journey they may feel extra vulnerable at this time. They may have had progesterone treatments as a way to support a potential pregnancy. Progesterone relaxes the smooth muscles of the uterus so as not to reject a fertilized egg.

Although there is no evidence at all that yoga could cause a miscarriage we can support with nourishing, building and spacious yoga sequences. I would continue the fluid circular flow from the ovulation section if a student feels connected to such a practice. The most important aspect of the yoga practice is how the student feels mentally and emotionally. If yoga makes them feel empowered, connected to their body, calm and relaxed then it can only be good for the potential pregnancy. If they feel anxious or worried, then it won't be.

As yoga teachers, we can educate ourselves so we are confident when we work with someone trying to conceive. We can learn pregnancy yoga. If someone is on an assisted fertility journey we can do some research and ask them questions too. No one expects us to know everything about everything. It is okay to ask questions, and if we don't feel confident we can refer them to someone who can provide the right support.

CHAPTER 13

Rest, Relaxation and Rejuvenation

The concept of *rasāyana*

I want to talk further about a couple of *Āyurvedic* concepts called *ojas* and *rasāyana*. This is relevant in a time where people seek (and need) yoga, *yin* yoga, restorative yoga and yoga *nidra* for their mental and emotional wellbeing, for their nervous system and to relax and rejuvenate.

The menstrual cycle is a hormonal event. Stress and anxiety affect our hormones, including the menstrual cycle. Finding ways to regulate the nervous system could affect the hormones and therefore the menstrual cycle too. In *Āyurveda*, the nervous system is associated with *vāta doṣa*. If *vāta doṣa* is disturbed it will eventually affect *pitta* and *kapha* too. Knowing a bit about *vāta doṣa* and its connection to menstruation specifically, and the cycle in general, we can conclude that stress and anxiety also affect the cycle from an *Āyurvedic* perspective.

We need ways to soothe the nervous system and any aggravated *vāta doṣa*. This is what we will discuss in this chapter.

As yoga teachers, we never stop learning. This is why you picked up this book. If you are like me, you have tons of books on various aspects of health and wellbeing – on different physiological, anatomical and psychological topics as well as more spiritual and yoga-specific subjects.

We have seen an increase in publications and courses on trauma and trauma-informed yoga, on the polyvagal theory, the nervous system and mindfulness. Yoga *nidra*, *yin* and restorative yoga seem to be more popular than ever. This trend supports that we, as a population, feel a need to rest and relax. We and our students are experiencing the benefits of a yoga practice. Western research, popular science and the media offer us more information on how important it is to regulate our nervous system, have good sleep habits and understand and take care of our mental health.

In *Āyurveda*, this has always been important. There is a whole branch of *Āyurveda* dedicated to rejuvenation called *rasāyana*. According to the classic *Āyurvedic* text, the *Caraka-saṃhitā*, someone undergoing *rasāyana* 'attains longevity, memory, intellect, freedom from diseases, youth, excellent lustre, complexion and voice', as well as 'respect and brilliance and a sharp memory'. It is important to note that this relates to specific treatments and herbs for patients suitable for these procedures. It also highlights just how important nourishing rejuvenating is in *Āyurvedic* healthcare.

Nourishing ojas

One of the main concepts when it comes to rejuvenation is the concept of *ojas*. We touched on the concepts of *ojas*, *tejas* and *prāṇa* in Chapter 3 where we introduced *Āyurveda*. But it is worth diving a little deeper into *ojas* as we discuss how our health and wellbeing rely on rest and being able to relax. *Ojas* is difficult to translate but we can refer to it as immunity, although that doesn't quite encompass all that it is. We say it is like nectar or *soma*. It is sweet and golden like honey and ghee (clarified butter).

Ojas is so important that, according to *Caraka*, 'if *ojas* is destroyed, the human being will also perish'. We have a superior type of *ojas* which is located in the heart. There are eight drops of this honey-like nectar here. Our life depends on these eight drops. When they perish, so will our life. The other more ordinary type of *ojas* constitutes all the seven bodily tissues or *dhātus*. If the *dhātus* are well and healthy, so is our *ojas*.

Someone with strong *ojas* will rarely get ill compared to someone with weak *ojas* who will easily get affected by potential disease-causing factors.

Of course, no system works alone. *Ojas* is determined by our *agni* or digestive fire and the relationship to *tejas* and *prāṇa*. This is often why we talk about *Āyurveda* and yoga being sister sciences. They complement each other. And we appreciate that yoga is a way of life, a philosophy and spiritual practice, not just an exercise programme. We need health in body, mind and spirit.

Ojas and the *doṣas*

Let's look at how the *doṣas* can influence *ojas*.

Pitta doṣa

Pitta is hot, sharp, penetrating, oily, greasy and fast. Anything we do, think, feel and eat with those qualities increase *pitta*. *Pitta*'s qualities as the refined *tejas* are essential for healthy *ojas*, but we can imagine how excess *pitta* can burn out and dry our *ojas*.

In the *pitta* part of the cycle, the luteal phase, we may experience more anger and irritability than usual. This is often due to excess *pitta*. Excess *pitta* reduces the quality of *ojas*. High *pitta doṣa* is generally due to lifestyle. Spicy food, alcohol, excess exercise, stress and running around too much can increase *pitta*. If you or any of your students are type-A personalities with a full diary and constant activities, and the only way you wind down is through a glass or two of red wine (*pitta* increasing) or through hardcore exercise, *ojas* will also be depleted. It is a vicious circle. We need time to reset and rejuvenate our *ojas*.

Yoga can also become depleting, especially when we refer to yoga as exercise. Hot yoga, for example, increases *pitta*. Excess heat dries out our *dhātus* (bodily tissues) and our *ojas*. A very dynamic power yoga session can do the same. Even a loud strenuous *ujjâyî prāṇayāma* can be excessively heating and depleting.

If someone tries too hard or pushes themselves too much it depletes the *ojas*.

Pitta people and people living in environments that increase *pitta doṣa*, such as big busy cities, need time to restore, cool and calm down. They need to replenish their *ojas*. In our yoga class, we do this by offering space to soothe the nervous system, to connect with the breath, slow down through movement and give permission to simply be and rest. This will help them avoid burnout and self-medicating through alcohol and being busy for the sake of feeling productive. Be mindful that *pitta* people might find it challenging to sit in meditation, slow-moving flows or be in a more *yin*-style *āsana* without striving or pushing themselves.

I had one such *pitta* person tell me that her family encouraged her to keep coming to yoga. They felt she was much calmer and more pleasant when she had a regular practice. It's a ripple effect for not just the individual but their relationships with family, friends and colleagues.

We know that stress and adrenalin influence our hormones and can affect the menstrual cycle. During the late luteal phase, this can manifest as any of the *pitta*-related symptoms such as premenstrual tension, anger, irritability, feeling hot and bothered. These symptoms are also associated with the perimenopause. Offering restorative, relaxing, nourishing and cooling yoga can be the antidote to excess *pitta* at any time in the cycle, during the perimenopause and beyond.

Vāta doṣa

Vāta doṣa is dry, cold, light, mobile, subtle, rough and irregular. If we have an irregular lifestyle and travel a lot, it increases *vāta doṣa.* Irregular meals have the same effect. Talking excessively, being on the computer and any kind of overstimulation can also increase *vāta.* When the weather is dry, windy or changeable it can increase *vāta.* Basically, *vāta* has the complete opposite qualities to *ojas*, which is nourishing, building, smooth, soft and sweet like nectar. If *vāta doṣa* is too high it will dry out and decrease *ojas.*

Vāta doṣa is the element of air, or wind, and space. When the wind blows, it dries what it comes in contact with. Too much *vāta* dries out the juicy, slightly oily or unctuous *ojas. Vāta* is rough and *ojas* is smooth.

The subtle aspect of *vāta* is *prāṇa. Prāṇa* and *tejas* together create healthy *ojas.* David Frawley (2012, p.95) explains how '*tejas* and *ojas*...connect to the solar and lunar currents, the *pingala* and *ida* of *yogic* thought. *Prāṇa* is the background force behind *tejas* and *ojas*, at once their result and their origin'. When we practise *prāṇayāma* or meditations on the lunar and solar energy, such as *nāḍīśōdhana* (alternate nostril breathing), we work with these three subtle aspects of *prāṇa*, *tejas* and *ojas.* We are trying to find equilibrium, between the solar and lunar, the right and the left, *Puruṣa* and *Prakṛti*, the non-gendered masculine and feminine energies.

Vāta can be the most challenging *doṣa* to balance because it is so irregular and erratic. There is not a lot of substance. To balance *vāta doṣa* we need to reduce *vāta*-increasing activities and habits.

Any movement is due to *vāta. Vāta* is mobility. The movement of the many thoughts in the mind is perhaps the most challenging aspect to balance. *Vāta doṣa* thinks a lot. This is why *vāta* people are prone to anxiety and insomnia. Too much thinking is exhausting. There is an increasing number of people reporting symptoms of anxiety and insomnia and it's become a health crisis. The NHS (National Health Service 2018) reports that 5 per cent of the UK population suffers from a generalized anxiety disorder. I believe the figure is much higher than that.

The downward movement of *vāta*, *apāna vāyu*, is prominent at menstruation. If *vāta* is disturbed, the menstrual phase and any symptoms around the period will be affected.

In Chapter 8 on *Āyurvedic* physiology, we mentioned that menstruation is a natural *raktamokṣa*, or bloodletting, treatment. This process can be a part of *pañchakarma*, or a cleansing practice. When someone undergoes a detoxifying and potentially depleting *pañchakarma* or an intense cleanse in *Āyurveda* they also undergo a nourishing and rejuvenating *rasāyana* treatment afterwards. This is to build up the *ojas* and any depletion in the body or mind post-cleanse. It could be through treatments such as *abhyanga* (oil massage) or oils baths as well as diet and herbs. If this is not done properly, the patient is weak and prone to imbalances or disease again. In the West, we might have heard of or tried *pañchakarma*, but many forget about the just as important practice of *rasāyana*.

From this angle, menstruation is slightly depleting although not like a full detox, cleansing programme or *pañchakarma*. We mustn't deplete ourselves even more through *vāta*-increasing activities. It is important to increase *ojas* and enjoy more nourishing practices to rebalance again.

Increased *vāta* can benefit by restoring and rejuvenating through connecting with the breath to calm the mind. *Vāta* is wind, air and space. *Prāṇa* is connected to *vāta*. *Prāṇa* is the lifeforce. It is energy. We practise *āsana*, *prāṇayāma* and meditation to support and balance *prāṇa*. Part of *rasāyana*, or rejuvenation, and supporting *ojas* is to practise breath awareness. Using the breath, we can regulate *prāṇa* and calm *vāta* to quiet the mind. This in turn can support *ojas*. Although we don't want to manipulate the movement of *apāna vāyu* during menstruation, breath awareness is useful during this phase. The rest of the month we can also enjoy *prāṇayāma* to soothe the nervous system and *vāta doṣa*. If the mind is too busy we, as teachers, can guide our students through meditations, breathing techniques, focused awareness and yoga *nidra*.

Kapha doṣa

Kapha doṣa is cold, wet, heavy, stable, solid, unctuous and slow. The positive and balanced qualities of *kapha* are very similar to those of *ojas*. But if there is excess *kapha* and it influences *ojas*, it becomes heavy, dull and slow. It can cause stagnation and accumulation. This can build up and increase *kapha doṣa* further, like a vicious circle. Once again, it is about finding balance.

We do not want to increase *kapha* to increase *ojas*, but rather find ways to support *ojas* through a healthy, balanced lifestyle. We can consider the connection between *prāṇa*, *tejas* and *ojas* again. Supporting the refined, more subtle qualities.

Finding the balance of movement and rest

As always this is about balance. Many yoga practices in the vein of women's yoga, menstrual yoga, menopause yoga or womb yoga only focus on restorative practices. While it's true that most of us need to rest more, we also need strength and mobility. We need focused rest and we need mindful movement for our physical, mental, emotional and energetic wellbeing, not distracting ourselves by *vāta*-increasing activities such as flicking through Netflix or scrolling on social media. Yoga is perfect for calming the mind and soothing or regulating the nervous system. We know this. There is plenty of research on yoga and wellbeing.

Mental and emotional stress causes physiological reactions in the body, including a hormonal response which in turn influences the menstrual cycle. Feeling run down can also cause havoc with the cycle. Rest and rejuvenation through a yoga practice may help to support the hormonal balance and the *doṣas*, and increase *ojas*. This will have a positive effect on the menstrual cycle.

I am convinced that breathing properly can alleviate many menstrual cycle complaints. How we breathe affects our stress levels and the hormones associated with stress and anxiety. Hormones affect other hormones, including those influencing the menstrual cycle. The nervous system, including the vagus nerve, is affected by our breathing pattern. The vagus nerve innervates the ovaries and uterus. Our womb and *yoni* are affected by and affect the nervous system. Finally, the respiratory and pelvic diaphragm are intrinsically connected – they move together – and pelvic floor health affects the pelvic organs. *Yogāsana* is a way to relieve physical tension, which again affects how we breathe.

Everything is connected.

CHAPTER 14

Yoga for Specific Complaints

We may have been told that period pain and cramps are normal. They are not, but they are common. We are not physiologically meant to experience pain and cramps, although we may experience some sensation. Remember *Āyurveda*'s very specific descriptions of the perfect period: the colour of the blood should be bright red like that of rabbit blood or a red lotus flower. It shouldn't stain clothes or have a foul smell (although it will have an aroma). It should be clot-free. The amount, according to the *Āyurvedic* classics, is four *anjalees*. One *anjali* is the amount you can have in your own cupped hands. An ideal period would last three to five days, and it shouldn't be painful.

Many of the symptoms and complaints are so common we think they are normal. I use the word common unless something is a normal physiological process or symptom.

In this chapter, we will look at some of the most common complaints, in alphabetical order.

Acne

Western perspective

As hormones drop just before the menstrual phase, we can experience more outbreaks. Oestrogen, as well as progesterone, can be quite good for the skin. Progesterone rises in the luteal phase, increasing sebum production which can cause the skin to become oilier. For some, this is a great moisturiser for their dry skin. For others, it creates clogged-up pores, which can cause bacteria growth, leading to inflammation and outbreaks.

Āyurvedic perspective

Skin issues are generally thought of as manifestations of deep-rooted issues often related to our digestion. Most of the *doṣas* are involved. *Vāta* might have slowed down our digestion and ability to eliminate. This can cause *āma* (toxins), which eventually manifest in the skin as breakouts. *Pitta* and the relationship to the blood tissue of *rakta* can cause inflammation and heat, leading to irritated, hot and angry skin. *Kapha*'s oily quality can cause excess sebum production. And then we have the hormonal rollercoaster of changes through the cycle.

Acne needs a personalized solution but looking at digestion and making sure we eliminate well with proper bowel movements is a good start. Then we need to calm down excess heat and fire and look at balancing *pitta doṣa* and *rakta dhātu* (blood tissue). It needs to be a very individualized treatment plan.

Yoga practices for acne

Although there aren't any specific yoga poses for hormonal acne, we can look at it from an *Āyurvedic* perspective and there are practices we can include throughout the month.

Good digestion is paramount from an *Āyurvedic* perspective. Include ways to create good blood circulation and movement to the abdomen and therefore the intestines to support digestion and elimination. *Sūryanamaskāra* (sun salutations) and *vinyāsa* flow can be good to increase stimulation. Any core work such as plank pose variations where you hug one knee to the chest kindles the digestive and core fire. The same applies to crow pose, *bakāsana*.

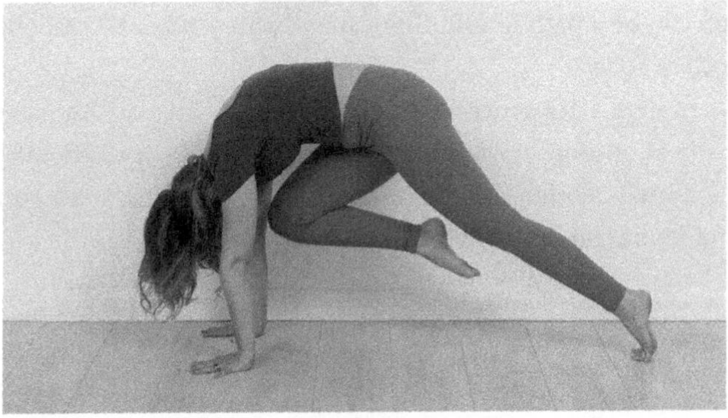

Plank pose variations hugging one knee to the chest using the core

Many yoga teachers refer to twists to detox the body. Although twists may not actually detox, they are effective in exercising the abdomen, almost like an abdominal massage. In this way, they can help digestion and release *āma*. Another excellent exercise is the classic *pawanmuktāsana* (wind-releasing) sequence from the Bihar School of yoga tradition. Lie supine hugging one knee to the chest while inhaling, release on the exhale, then do the same with the other leg, release and finally hug both knees to the chest and release. This variation is also recommended for anyone with excess *vāta*, especially manifested in the abdomen as wind.

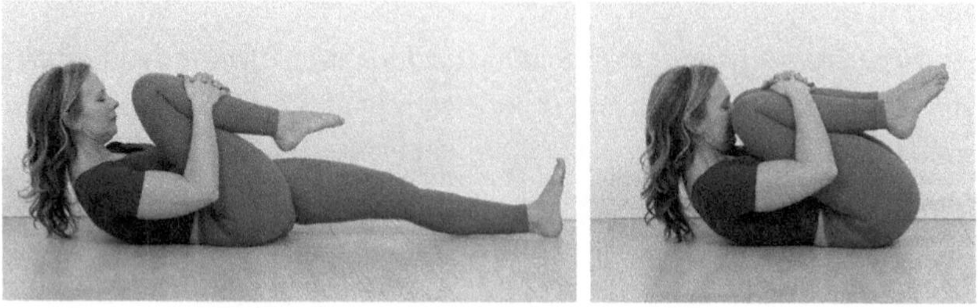

Pawanmuktāsana or the wind-releasing sequence

If *vāta doṣa* doesn't flow properly it may cause obstruction, and excess heat or *pitta* will rise upwards. This could be another reason for menstrual or premenstrual acne. Looking at digestion, we support the movement of *vāta*, as well as stimulating any slow and stagnated *kapha*. Now we need to calm any hot and fiery *pitta* which can cause redness, inflammation and irritation of the skin.

Cooling breaths like *sheetali prāṇayāma* calms *pitta doṣa*. *Nāḍīśodhana* (alternate nostril breathing) is also balancing. Embracing meditation and relaxation can be a path to mindfulness and a less inflamed response to the experience of acne.

Forward bends are generally calming when practised with patience. So, include any soothing forward bends you like, such as *paschimottanāsana* (seated forward bends), *upavishta konāsana* (wide-angle seated forward bend) and *janu sirsāsana* (head-to-knee forward bend).

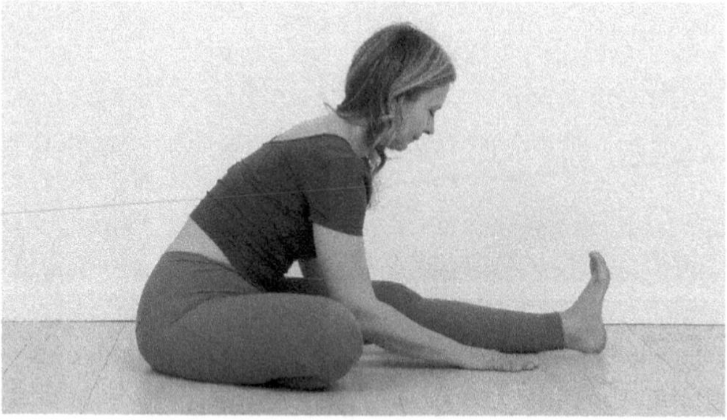

Janu sirsāsana. Use props or modifications when appropriate

Standing forward bends create more blood circulation to the head and we can imagine how this may support healthy skin tissue as well. *Uttanāsana* (standing forward bend) or *prasarita padottanāsana* (wide-legged forward bend) are great for this.

Inversions can be calming as well as bringing plenty of blood circulation to the head, keeping the skin healthy. *Śīrṣāsana* (headstand) and *sālamba-sarvāṅgāsana* (shoulderstand) can both be meditative and calming for the mind and for *vāta* and *pitta doṣa*. Choose inversions appropriate for your students.

Bloating, swelling and water retention

Western perspective

Abdominal bloating can be due to changes in the digestion as progesterone rises in the mid-luteal phase then sharply drops just before the menstrual phase. Progesterone can slow things down. It can slow digestion and therefore cause constipation and bloating.

But bloating in the premenstrual and menstrual phase is not just digestion. It is also about the fluids in the body affecting the feet, hands and breasts, for example. Research suggests that both estradiol (an oestrogen) and progesterone have important effects on body fluid and sodium regulation and, in effect, the potential for bloating (Stachenfeld 2008).

Āyurvedic perspective

Kapha doṣa is water and earth. *Kapha* is slow, accumulative and stagnant. We can associate water retention with *kapha doṣa*. Although the luteal and menstrual phase where we often experience swelling isn't associated with *kapha*, we can still get *kapha* symptoms.

We need to get *kapha* moving. Any active yoga movement and exercise is great for *kapha* and the lymphatic system.

Yoga practices for bloating

If the abdominal bloating is due to wind and excess *vāta*, the Bihar School of yoga tradition's classic *pawanmuktāsana* sequence, as mentioned previously, is perfect: lying supine, hug each knee to the chest one at a time, and then both knees. Part of the series is also moving all the joints: rotating the ankles and wrists, flexing and extending the knees and elbows. Although it is translated as the 'wind-releasing' exercise, it works well for fluid retention and *kapha* too.

Retention and stagnation need flow and movement. Dynamic *vinyāsa* yoga flows are great for this. In the section about acne, we discussed the importance of digestion and the same principles and poses apply here for abdominal bloating. Enjoy lots of twists and activate the core.

For swollen ankles, inversions and *viparīta karaṇī* (legs-up-the-wall) are great too. This supports the lymphatic flow back to the lymph nodes and potentially reduces the swelling in the lower legs and feet.

Clots

Western perspective

During menstruation, the uterus sheds the uterine lining. This causes the capillaries to break and bleed. If this happens anywhere else in the body, such as if you cut your finger or graze your knee, the body will naturally respond by blood coagulation trying to stop bleeding. This essentially solidifies the blood and eventually forms a protective scab.

However, during menstruation, the body produces anticoagulants so that the blood can be released as a period. If the flow is heavy, the anticoagulants may not be able to keep up and the blood tissue and uterine lining will start to coagulate, forming clots.

Passing a large clot through the cervix and out through the vaginal canal can cause extreme pain. It can also be associated with heavy flow and cramps as the uterus contracts to expel the clots. There can be other underlying causes that need to be investigated.

Āyurvedic perspective

Clots are generally associated with heavy menstruation, which in *Āyurveda* could be caused by either *kapha* or *pitta*. However, most imbalances start with some kind of *vāta* vitiation. When you look at your student you may notice the general qualities associated with either of these *doṣas* and then customize the yoga practice accordingly.

When heavy periods are associated with clots it's a manifestation of stagnation, accumulation and build-up, which are all *kapha*, although it also involves movement and flow (*vāta*) as well as the blood tissue (*rakta dhātu*) associated with *pitta*. As always in *Āyurveda*, we look at the individual and their lifestyle, not just the symptoms. Clots can be something that may happen just once in a while or be a regular occurrence. This is why it is so important to be tracking the menstrual cycle so we can notice these patterns.

Yoga practices for clots

When *vāta doṣa* creates an imbalance it lays the foundation for the other *doṣas* to shift too. Any calming practice is suitable for both *vāta* and *pitta* individuals. Focusing on warmth and breathing will help balance *vāta* as well as *kapha*. Grounding practices with some fluidity and awareness of the pelvis are good for our pelvic organs, menstrual cycle and all the *doṣas*.

During the menstrual phase, gentle movements and stretches are typically encouraged. If someone has heavy periods and cramping as the uterus tries to expel clots, they may just want to curl up on the sofa with a hot water bottle. The warmth from the hot water bottle is soothing for vitiated *vāta* and *kapha* as well as for the muscles of the uterus. However, if the cause is more *pitta*, a cool compress might be more effective. I also like gentle rocking seated in a crossed-legged position during cramping, maybe with a gentle *ujjâyî prāṇayāma* to focus and calm the breath and as a pathway to soothe any unnecessary tension and contraction in the body.

Bālāsana (child's pose) is maybe the most comfortable position, but opening up with a supported *setubandhāsana* (bridge pose) and *suptabaddhakoṇāsana* (reclined cobbler's pose) can also be useful.

After the period, it is good to create some stimulation for the pelvic area. Follow the suggestions for the follicular phase during this time, focusing on the warming and activating *kapālabhāti* (skull-shining breath) and *bhastrikā* (bellows breath), the twisting and forward bends with some compression of the abdomen (e.g. roll up a blanket and place at the lower abdomen in seated forward bends). *Malāsana* (squatting) is a way to encourage *apāna vāyu* as well as opening the hips. *Malāsana* is not recommended during the menstrual phase but can be practised at any other time in the cycle.

These suggestions all support the movement to break up stagnation in the pelvis which can accumulate and create clots. For this reason, you may also want to consider the suggestions from the follicular phase through to the late luteal phase too. If there is a sense of depletion, stress and vitiated *pitta*, embrace the cooling and calming practises discussed in Chapter 13 on rest, relaxation and rejuvenation.

Cramps (see painful periods)

Endometriosis

Western perspective

The endometrium is the inner layer, or lining, of the uterus. The endometrial layer is shed during the period and slowly builds up again through the cycle. In endometriosis, the endometrium (or similar tissues) starts to grow outside the uterus, and as it's not in the uterus, it can't be released during menstruation.

It is unclear why this happens. What we do know is that it can be extremely painful and that symptoms can vary from person to person. Symptoms include abdominal pain and lower backache, which becomes worse during menstruation. Pain during sex is another issue. Feeling nauseous, experiencing diarrhoea or constipation are just some of the other complaints.

From a Western perspective, there is currently no cure for endometriosis and symptoms are treated, although it can be challenging to find the perfect solution for the individual.

Āyurvedic perspective

Kapha doṣa is involved, with its qualities of building up, accumulation, growth and stagnation, but as the growth of the endometrial lining is outside its normal place (the uterus), *vāta doṣa* is also involved. Instead of *apāna vāyu* moving down and out, it is flowing in the wrong direction. The endometrium, or the energy of the endometrium, is not building up in its correct place, the uterus, and instead *vāta doṣa* is pushing it outside the uterine cavity. Another quality of vitiated *vāta doṣa* is pain. Endometriosis is painful. Endometriosis is also thought of as being an oestrogen-dependent inflammatory disease which corresponds with *kapha doṣa* (Lin *et al.* 2018).

We can consider that *vāta doṣa* is a potential initiator, pushing *pitta* and *kapha* out of place. It is possible that *āma*, or undigested material, is part of the process too. This doesn't need to be digestive issues, but could be a build up of *āma* in other ways too, even mental *āma*. The first step is to encourage *vāta* balance and for *apāna vāyu* to move in its correct direction. We also want to break up any accumulated and stagnated energy and create flow again.

This condition can become a vicious circle. The cause can be of *vāta* origin, which can bring about pain and anxiety. This aggravates *vāta* even more, which then causes more pain, more anxiety and potentially continues to displace *pitta* and *kapha*, causing more endometriosis and pain. This is another reason to calm down *vāta doṣa* in our approach.

Yoga practices for endometriosis

There is some evidence that yoga can be useful for people with endometriosis, both reducing pelvic pain and improving quality of life. One study concluded, 'Women said they had identified a relationship between pain management and breathing techniques (*prāṇayāma*) learned in yoga and that breathing increased their ability to be introspective, which relieved pain' (Gonçalves, Barros & Bahamondes 2017; Gonçalves *et al.* 2016).

The priority is to allow the flow of *apāna vāyu*. This means we avoid anything that may cause *apāna* to be disturbed. I would eliminate or reduce inversions, strong *mūlabandha*, Kegel exercises, or any excessive core work. This is because they either manipulate *apāna vāyu* in the wrong direction or cause contraction in the area in the case of extreme core work. Some core work is good for the blood and lymphatic circulation in the pelvis, pelvic organs and digestion, but the focus is to create flow and movement rather than contraction.

I am passionate about pelvic floor health and we all need to be aware of these muscles, and from an energetic perspective too. Just as we can have tightness and constrictions in our shoulders, our pelvic floor can also be tight. Work to create mobility at the pelvic floor rather than just engaging or tightening the muscles. We need to learn to relax the pelvic diaphragm. Again, think of circulation and allowing *apāna vāyu* to release.

Consider the practices we did in the late luteal phase with the emphasis on letting go, as well as the menstrual phase yoga. These are beneficial for endometriosis. During menstruation, adhere to the yoga suggested for the menstrual phase to encourage *apāna*.

Here are some of my suggested poses from these two phases: pelvic rocking and circling in a seated pose or combined into standing flows. *Pawanmuktāsana* for the abdomen, where you lie on the back bringing one knee to the chest, release, then bring the other knee, release and finally bring both knees, continuing for three to five rounds. Add backbends, forward bends and twists into the sequence, with a focus on creating flow and stimulation around the lower abdomen and pelvis. *Malāsana* (yogīc squat) is the ultimate *apāna vāyu*-encouraging yoga pose practised outside the menstrual phase.

Also, consider any meditation practice or *prāṇayāma* you offer. Many meditations are about drawing the energy upwards. Although we may want that for our spiritual awakening, we need to be grounded in our physical body first. Our body needs to be healthy and pain-free. I would discourage any practices where there is an intense focus on raising the energy; instead, enjoy body-centred and body-positive practices.

Fatigue

Western perspective

It is quite common to feel fatigued just before and during the first few days of the period. This is caused by a drop in oestrogen. You may remember that oestrogen is a feel-good hormone. It is at its lowest just before and around the first days of the menstrual phase. Another happiness hormone is serotonin and this affects our energy levels too. It is thought that people with low serotonin or a drop of serotonin experience fatigue at this time. This is often connected with the decrease in oestrogen at the end of the luteal phase (Hall & Steiner 2013).

Another reason for fatigue during the menstrual phase can be heavy bleeding causing low haemoglobin levels and a low iron count. See the section on heavy periods if this is the cause.

Āyurvedic perspective

Tiredness and lethargy are usually associated with *kapha doṣa* or a *tāmasic* energy. We also get fatigued if we are run down. A *pitta* person gets burned out. A *vāta* person gets overwhelmed and then exhausted. *Kapha* people can have a tendency to feel heavy and low. If we are already weak, tired, overwhelmed, burned out or exhausted, this will be highlighted at the late luteal and early menstrual phases of the cycle. This is why menstrual cycle tracking and menstrual cycle awareness is so important. We get to know our patterns.

The shift just before and the first few days of the menstrual phase are sensitive times. A lot is going on with the hormones, in the physical body and of course the *doṣic* changes, and all of this affects the mind, emotions and energetic being.

Vāta doṣa is prominent. *Vāta* is air and space and is easily distracted. There is not a lot of substance or endurance and this can cause fatigue. The main energy is *apāna vāyu*, which is the downward and outward movement of *prāṇa*. The body is in *raktamokṣa* mode. The solution is an individual approach to create balance through the whole cycle, and a focus on rest.

As you are reading through this book you may have noticed how conditioned we are to live a continuous, linear lifestyle with no consideration for our hormonal, *doṣic*, cyclic or energetic shifts. *Āyurvedic* lifestyle and menstrual cycle awareness is not just about the yoga routine and exercise we commit to through the month. It is also how we approach life, work, family commitments, food, diet, activities and most importantly our own expectations of how we 'should' perform in life. Remembering to take time to rest before becoming fatigued, burned out or overwhelmed is part of that awareness.

Yoga practices for fatigue

Probably the most important thing to look at is the full cycle. How is the practice during the follicular phase and around ovulation? More importantly, has there been space to slow down and embrace rest too? It is easy to exert oneself through the cycle, especially in the follicular and ovulatory phases, and to then crash around menstruation. We need to take time to rest throughout the cycle.

Fatigue can be part of PMS symptoms or be felt during the first few days of the cycle. In either case, we want to look at allowing rest and rejuvenation. This corresponds with what we suggest in Chapter 12 on yoga during the menstrual phase.

If a *kapha*-dominant person is tired it may be the general heaviness, slowness or potentially any *tāmasic* tendencies that are exacerbated. In this case, focus on *sattvic* qualities in the practice. A *kapha* person needs encouragement to keep moving and stay active. Even if it's just a gentle walk or a short daily routine of a few yoga poses or *sūryanamaskāra* (sun salutations).

If the person is dominantly *vāta*, we can offer a slow, nourishing, grounding, steady and warming yoga session aimed at calming the mind and the nervous system specifically. Slow deep breathing such as the three-part breath and diaphragmatic breathing is good, as is the balancing *nāḍīśōdhana* (alternate nostril breathing). *Brāmari* (bumblebee) breath is excellent to calm down the mind.

If the lifestyle and tendencies are more *pitta* dominant, we focus on cooling and calming down. *Sheetali prāṇayāma* (cooling breath) cools and soothes the hot, fiery and burned-out *pitta* mind. Encourage a seated meditation to be still and calm. *Pitta* needs to be reminded of the importance of rest and rejuvenation, which was explained in detail in Chapter 13.

If the body is fatigued, we need to rest and rejuvenate. It's okay to do nothing, and it's okay not to practise yoga or exercise every day. If it becomes a stressful event or depleting, then stop for a few days – or even longer. Or embrace a more lunar meditative yoga such as *yin*, restorative yoga or *soma vinyāsa* as we described in Chapter 13.

Fertility

Western perspective

Being fertile is having a healthy cycle. We can think of the menstrual cycle as the fifth vital sign of health (the others being body temperature, blood pressure, pulse and respiration rate). It shows us if there are hormonal imbalances and it indicates our stress levels too. It is not necessarily about wanting to conceive.

You are likely to have clients trying to conceive asking for support, which is why I include it here. Fertility is not just about the female reproductive system. Sperm quality and quantity are important factors and often less invasive to investigate. However, here we are focusing on a healthy cycle. There are numerous reasons why it can be challenging to become pregnant. Many will come to you with the diagnosis of 'unexplained fertility', meaning there is no known medical reason as to why they haven't conceived.

Āyurvedic perspective

The *Āyurvedic* classics discuss in detail how to prepare for pregnancy for both parents-to-be. This includes herbs, lifestyle and *pañchakarma* (detox), as well as the specific ages for both partners and even the best time and sex positions. In the *Caraka-saṃhitā* it says, 'O Lord! Among human beings, women are the excellent raison d'etre of progeny,' and it goes on to discuss the importance of the aetiology (origin), signs, symptoms and treatments of gynaecological 'disorders for the welfare of humanity'. Perhaps this is the reason why there is a great deal of emphasis on gynaecology and menstrual wellness in *Āyurveda*.

I was fortunate to be an apprentice in *Āyurvedic* hospitals in India where they did exceptional work and research in fertility. This is still an area of expertise in *Āyurvedic* medicine with specialist consultants and departments.

In this book, we focus on the menstrual cycle. A healthy regular cycle is a sign of general health and wellbeing. In *Āyurveda*, we look at our lifestyle through the seasons, the weather, the external environment and our individual constitution. We also look at how we live according to the inner seasons – the menstrual cycle. Using the principles in this book and applying them to our general lifestyle is the first step to menstrual and fertility health.

Endometriosis, polycystic ovary syndrome and amenorrhoea (not menstruating) can all affect fertility. In these cases, look up the individual complaint.

Yoga practices for fertility

There will be students asking for yoga to support the fertility journey, which is why I added the 'trying to conceive' subheading into the sections on yoga during each phase of the cycle.

As yoga teachers, our expertise is yoga. We can refer to fertility experts within the medical community, *Āyurvedic* doctors and practitioners or other healthcare providers when it comes to diet, medication, herbs and treatments. As we know, yoga can be an amazing complementary therapy to other interventions.

Yoga can support our mental and emotional wellbeing, reducing stress and anxiety. From a yoga perspective, we create balance and encourage *sattva guṇa* of bliss rather than being drawn into a *rajasic* state of too much stress or anger, or being *tāmasic* with the tendencies of inertia and feeling low. In *Āyurveda*, we aim to create *doṣic* balance not just in the physical body but also emotionally and mentally.

Coming to yoga to find that space of calm and ease can be a great support on the fertility journey – and we can use the guidance in this book for a healthy fertile cycle.

Fibroids

Western perspective

Fibroids in or around the uterus are very common, with one in three people having them according to the NHS (National Health Service 2018). Fibroids are non-cancerous growths and can be of various sizes. Some people will never know they have fibroids and have no symptoms at all, but they can grow large and cause complications such as heavy and painful periods, as well as abdominal pain, pain during intercourse and constipation. So, it's worth being checked out.

There is no clear aetiology or cause for fibroids. There might be a link to high oestrogen but the research is contradictory and scant. There is also no treatment or cure. The symptoms may be treated, there are drugs helping to reduce their size, and potentially surgery could be required.

Āyurvedic perspective

Growths are mentioned in *Āyurvedic* literature as *granthi* and there are various *Āyurvedic* treatments and approaches for these. All the *doṣas* are involved in this specific growth. *Vāta* is involved as the pelvis is the home of *vāta doṣa*. *Kapha doṣa* is about growth and solidity. There is some *pitta doṣa* involvement too, as it is connected to hormones and blood or *rakta*. Again, this is connected to *dhātus* or the tissues of the body, specifically blood (*rakta*), muscle (*mamsa*) and fat (*meda*) (Dhiman 2014).

We want to reduce excess *vāta* and *kapha*. In *Āyurveda*, we would do this with herbs, diet and body treatments, but we can also consider how our yoga practice can support the process.

Yoga practices for fibroids

Vāta and *kapha* both like warmth. They can both have challenges with digestion, which is one of the pillars of health. If we don't digest well, we create *āma* (undigested material), causing toxic reactions in *Āyurveda*.

Creating warmth, stimulation and flow in the lower abdomen can support digestion but also encourage flow and circulation to the pelvic organs such as the uterus where the fibroids grow.

Breathing practices such as *kapālabhāti* (skull-shining breath) and *bhastrikā* (bellows breath) stimulate the lower abdomen to strengthen the digestive fire. They are also generally good for *kapha doṣa*.

I would include lots of twists in the yoga practice to stimulate and massage the abdomen and the digestive system. The same with forward bends, perhaps adding extra compression to the lower abdomen. Backbends are often recommended for pelvic and menstrual health in yoga literature and are a group of poses often used in research on painful periods in general. The focus is to give energy and warmth to the lower abdomen, the intestines and the uterus.

Heavy periods or heavy menstrual bleeding (menorrhagia)

Western perspective

This is perhaps one of the most common menstrual complaints and can impact a person's life significantly, for example not wanting to leave their home in case they bleed through clothing, not wanting to socialize or do exercise, having to put extra towels on the bed in case they bleed through during the night. Aside from it being uncomfortable, it can also cause so much blood loss it leads to anaemia.

According to the NHS (National Health Service 2021a), heavy menstrual bleeding is defined as losing 80ml or more during the menstrual phase, having periods that last longer than seven days, or both. This could mean you change your period product every hour, are bleeding through your clothes or bed linen or need to use two types of period products together. It is often accompanied by larger clots. There can be a feeling that the blood is gushing out, making the prospect of going out or even moving at all very tricky.

There can be underlying reasons such as fibroids, polycystic ovaries, other uterine abnormalities or endometriosis, so it is good to have a check-up with the GP and potentially get a scan.

Many people with heavy periods will not have any of the underlying conditions mentioned above. Heavy menstrual bleeding can be managed through hormones, using birth control such as the pill or the coil, which shut down the natural cycle and can either make the symptoms worse or better. Non-hormonal options are limited to tranexamic acid, which helps coagulation and thereby reduces the bleed, or potentially a hysterectomy. Iron supplements may also be prescribed.

The pattern of the menstrual cycle and the amount we bleed can change through our life and especially when we first start menstruating at menarche and as we enter perimenopause.

Āyurvedic perspective

Pitta being hot, sharp and penetrating is often associated with heavy periods. *Pitta* also has a connection with *rakta dhātu*, the blood tissue. In *Āyurveda*, *pitta*-dominant people may generally have heavier periods.

Kapha doṣa is slow, accumulative and heavy. This includes the manifestation of menses, which can also be heavy and long.

But, we are all unique beings and there can be several causative factors. It is worth bearing in mind that the pelvis is the seat of *vāta doṣa* and *vāta* is often the initiator of creating imbalances for the other *doṣas*. *Vāta* is movement and flow so although *vāta* periods are generally light, *vāta* can cause havoc, with the other *doṣas* and *dhātus* being the root cause for heavy menstrual bleeding.

Heavy flow can be hormonal (e.g. perimenopause). Hormones are often related to *pitta doṣa* whereas change is *vāta*. It can be due to underlying causes such as abnormal growth as mentioned in the Western perspective.

Stress, burnout and exhaustion can be a factor. The body is overwhelmed and tired and there is not enough energy to support the functioning of the uterus, and *apāna vāyu*, during menses. There is a sense of depletion. *Vāta doṣa* has become vitiated, either due to *vāta*-increasing activities of doing and thinking too much, not eating well, having very irregular meals, being out and about excessively, travelling and not taking time to rest; or perhaps due to *pitta* with its type-A personality of *doing* (all the time) rather than *being*, excessive exercise or increased alcohol and too much spicy and hot food.

Either way, calming down *vāta* and *pitta* in the body and mind by resting is essential. Even *kapha doṣa* people need calm and mindful rest. We need to replenish. And that is what yoga can bring: stillness without heaviness.

Yoga practices for heavy periods

Because periods are expressions of our general health and wellbeing in body and mind we need a full cycle approach. Consider the individual's *doṣas* and then apply the cyclical yoga approach for each of the phases of the menstrual cycle.

As mentioned above, it is important to find a way to rest and practise mindfulness. It is essential to rejuvenate and restore in *Āyurveda*. Yet, it's also important to create strength and a sense of 'clearing out' just after the menstrual phase. Find a balance through the cycle, to create strength in the body without exhaustion. And find ways to rest. This is not just about the yoga practice, it is about how we move through life. Perhaps through these principles we can find other ways to nourish a depleted body with wholesome foods and soulful interactions, to ease off the treadmill of the busyness of life.

Menstruation is *raktamokṣa* and it is a cleanse. During the menstrual phase, we want to practise *being* rather than *doing*. We want to rest, and if we practise yoga it should be more restorative or therapeutic. This is just as we would rest during any detox or cleanse.

If you or your students experience heavy periods, consider a practice to replenish and nourish. This means including yoga poses and practices such as *yin* style or restorative yoga. Also consider meditations, *prāṇayāma* and, if appropriate, yoga philosophy – spiritual practices and devotional yoga to nourish the soul. Don't just do this during the menstrual phase but emphasize these practices throughout the cycle.

When menstruating with a heavy flow, one might not want to move at all. Either it is just uncomfortable or there is a fear of leaking through the clothes. Resting is absolutely fine. We do not have to practise every day.

Viparīta karaṇī (legs-up-the-wall) or resting the lower legs on a chair may feel grounding and nourishing, as can *bālāsana* (child's pose) and supported forward bends, either seated or standing. A low supported *setubandhāsana* (bridge pose) can also give some relief. If the flow is very heavy it may feel uncomfortable to do any poses where the legs are wide apart or asymmetric. Focus on restoring with rest, including supported *shavāsana*, yoga *nidra* and gentle breathing.

Irregular periods (oligomenorrhea)

Western perspective

A regular period means you know approximately how long your cycle is and it is generally the same, although it might be a couple of days off sometimes. As an example, if your cycle is 23 days one month and then 35 days the next, it is irregular. This is common during puberty when the menstrual (and ovulatory) cycle begins, and during the perimenopause as we leave the cycles behind.

Irregular cycles could be a symptom of polycystic ovary syndrome, thyroid issues or extreme weight gain or weight loss. It can also manifest during stressful times. According to the NHS website (National Health Service 2021b), irregular periods are not a sign of a problem although it is recommended to see a doctor just in case.

Some medications can affect the cycle, including hormonal contraception which basically stops or changes your natural flow of hormones. There are some reports of changes to the menstrual cycle after Covid vaccinations but at the time of writing there is not enough sustainable data to offer any explanation or confirmation of this.

Āyurvedic perspective

Āyurveda looks at the menstrual cycle and menstruation itself as an expression of general health and wellbeing. If there are irregularities, it is a sign of an imbalance.

The menstrual cycle isn't just about periods. It is about having a healthy follicular phase, ovulation and luteal phase. All of these, along with menstruation, are signs of health. When we make notes of how we experience our cycle we might be able to find patterns. Even though the period can't be predicted there might be patterns of the follicular phase, maybe a sign of ovulation and an awareness of when the luteal phase begins.

If the period is early or late, there is something off with the follicular or luteal phase. Or perhaps we have cycles with no ovulation.

Most of us have experienced late or early periods outside puberty and the perimenopause. Usually, it happens in times of stress, grief, illness or significant life changes. These are events that increase *vāta doṣa*. *Vāta doṣa* has the quality of irregularity, and so our periods may be early or late. People with high *vāta* or a *vāta* lifestyle can experience very irregular periods.

Unless there is an underlying reason, the *Āyurvedic* approach is to reduce *vāta* in our lifestyle, diet and attitude. We looked at the individual *doṣas* in the introduction to *Āyurveda*. The qualities of *vāta* are dry, light, cold, rough, subtle, mobile and clear. We reduce those qualities in our food and routine and implement the opposites: finding a regular routine, sleeping and waking at the same time each day, eating warming slightly oily foods. Instead of moving continuously in body and mind, we try to find stillness and steadiness.

Yoga practices for irregular periods

We counteract irregularity with regularity. If there is awareness of where in the cycle the student is, we can use that to implement the general yoga guidelines for the different phases of the cycle.

However, regardless of where the person is in their cycle, we can focus on mindfulness, awareness, creating steadiness and getting grounded. These qualities are all *vāta* balancing. So even in the follicular phase, where we practise arm balances or core work, we can encourage steadiness of mind and body. In a creative flow, we can still create routine, balance and stability. We can always encourage our students to implement a daily routine of a few moments of *nāḍīśōdhana* (alternate nostril breathing) and maybe even a few yoga poses such as *vrkāsana* (tree pose) to find balance and get grounded, or a supported *setubandhāsana* (bridge pose) to open and stretch the lower abdomen and hips. Also consider an easy forward bend to calm the mind.

Most research on yoga for menstrual health is very general and looks at premenstrual symptoms or period pain. These are sometimes referred to as menstrual irregularities in research studies. However, one study (Jadhao 2019, p.1149) included irregular periods saying that yoga 'evoked a state of homeostasis, which perhaps helps to control anxiety, stress and several mood swings and improved the power of pain tolerance and other associated problems caused due to irregular menstruation. To summarize, yoga seems to be one of the illustrious ways to tackle menstrual delays'. This study included a starting prayer and Omkar recitation as well as *anuloma viloma* (alternate nostril breathing), *kapālabhāti* (skull-shining breath) and *bhastrikā* (bellows breath).

Another study (Kumaravelu & Das 2020, p.1764) looked at how 'yogīc practices balanced thyroid stimulating hormones among college girls suffering with irregular menstruation' with great success.

Many of the suggested yoga poses for menstrual irregularities as opposed to irregular periods include backbends such as *bhujangāsana* (cobra pose), *salabāsana* (locust pose) and *setubandhāsana* (bridge pose). *Pawanmukatāsana* (the Bihar School of Yoga's wind-releasing exercise sequence) also seems to be common in these studies on period complaints.

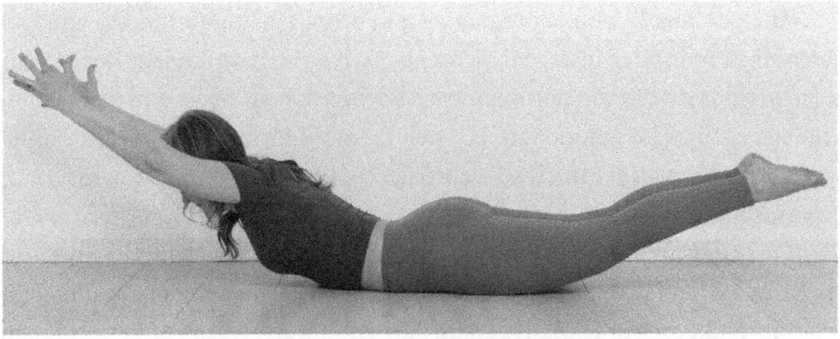

Variation of salabāsana. You can also offer other arm variations

Perhaps yoga as a regular practice supports general health and wellbeing, both physically and mentally, which also means a balanced menstrual cycle – and regularity is the antidote to excessive *vāta*.

No periods (amenorrhoea) and/or no ovulation

Western perspective

There are two types of amenorrhoea. According to the National Institute for Health and Care Excellence (NICE) (2020):

> primary amenorrhoea is defined as the failure to establish menstruation by 15 years of age in girls with normal secondary sexual characteristics (such as breast development), or by 13 years of age in girls with no secondary sexual characteristics. Secondary amenorrhoea is defined as the cessation of menstruation for 3–6 months in women with previously normal and regular menses, or for 6–12 months in women with previous oligomenorrhoea.

Oligomenorrhoea is defined as infrequent menstrual periods (fewer than six to eight periods per year). We would generally come across secondary amenorrhoea.

Although amenorrhoea is referring to not having a period, we need to look at the cycle as a whole. The menstrual cycle is not just about menstruation but also whether or not there is ovulation.

There can be several reasons why periods suddenly stop and these should be investigated. There can be hormonal reasons, including thyroid issues and polycystic ovary syndrome. Maybe there is no ovulation leading to menstruation. Some medications and treatments, including breast cancer protocols, affect the menstrual and ovulatory cycle.

The obvious reason is pregnancy and breastfeeding (although you can breastfeed and still ovulate and menstruate). We also have students with irregular periods due to the perimenopause, where ovulation and menstruation change again. The menopause is when there hasn't been a period for a full year. Stress and grief can cease menstruation for some time, as can excessive and insufficient weight.

One concept that's worth investigating when it comes to missing periods is RED-S or 'relative energy deficiency in sport'. This refers to insufficient caloric intake and/or excessive energy expenditure. It is seen not only in high performing athletes but also in anyone who doesn't get the nutrition they need, even for day-to-day activities (as we see in people with eating disorders). In this case, the student must get professional support to get enough nutrition, or with disordered eating, to gain understanding and recover.

Āyurvedic perspective

Anartava, or amenorrhoea, and most menstrual issues are caused or instigated by *vāta*, but there are variations and different reasons why an individual ceases to menstruate.

Caraka mentions the condition *arajaska* where *pitta* is displaced in the uterus causing *rakta dhātu* to become imbalanced, leading to amenorrhea. In this case, we need to reduce excess *pitta doṣa*. That means doing the opposite of *pitta* qualities throughout the cycle. No hot and fiery exercise, yoga or foods. Reduce alcohol. Perhaps through yogīc philosophy and spiritual teachings, find ways to be less attached to *doing* rather than *being* and to reduce anger and irritation. Connect with the higher self/the divine/nature rather than the ego. Favour cooling and calming qualities. Yoga is a great companion for *pitta* because it has a wealth of practices to calm and cool down the mind and to destress.

In *Āyurveda*, not eating enough, eating insufficient protein, carbohydrates and fats, eating irregularly and having too many cold and dry foods will increase *vāta doṣa*. *Vāta* is air and space, not solidity. In this case, we need to reduce *vāta doṣa* with routine, stability, oiliness, warmth and heaviness.

Another reason *vāta* aggravates is through mental stress and anxiety. If our mind and our general lifestyle are overwhelmed, our body goes into survival mode. Even if our stressors are not actual life-threatening emergencies, our body may believe they are due to the mental stress around the situations. If we are in a dangerous situation, ovulation and menstruation are not priorities and so the body may cease to have a regular cycle.

Vāta people are quick thinking and have plenty of creative ideas but can also have so many thoughts that it leads to anxiety and insomnia. They may forget to eat as they are so caught up in their thoughts and activities. In excess, *vāta* people are in their heads rather than being embodied. The energy is rising up rather than rooting down. In the yoga practice, we encourage *feeling* rather than *thinking*.

Pitta types are focused, dynamic, sharp and clear in their mindset when balanced. Imbalanced *pitta* is sensation-seeking and once they have a goal they won't stop until they get there (like high-performing athletes). This can mean they forget about their body, they don't take time to rest because they live on adrenalin and there is potential for anger and irritability. Just like *vāta*, they forget to listen to the body.

Because *kapha* can accumulate heaviness and stagnation in both body and mind, it can also stagnate and stop the menstrual cycle. Feeling depressed and low can be vitiated *kapha*, which can also lead to amenorrhea. Depression, grief, mental health issues and other *kapha* imbalances may lead to either weight gain or weight loss, which in turn affects the cycle. *Kapha* people need to move, and yoga is perfect for this with its mindful movement, breathing practices and spiritual components that may also support mental and emotional wellbeing.

I want to mention diet here as digestion is one of the pillars of health according to *Āyurveda*. Our food, our nourishment, creates our tissues (*dhātus*). Our diet affects both body and mind. It can create toxins, *āma*, as well as vitality, *ojas*. This is true for excess spicy hot sharp food, red meat and alcohol, which can aggravate *pitta doṣa*, affecting the blood tissue, *rakta dhātu*. It is also true when it comes to RED-S as mentioned above.

Whether the reason is primarily *vāta*, *pitta* or *kapha*, the underlying cause could stem from diet and certainly also from our mental health.

Yoga practices for amenorrhea

There is not one yoga protocol that works for everybody with amenorrhea or lack of ovulation as there are so many different causes. Obviously, pregnancy, postpartum recovery, postmenopause and certain medications are times when there will be no menstruation or ovulation and when no approach is needed to try to restore a cycle. In these cases, we can enjoy the cyclic yoga practices but align them with the moon. Menstrual phase yoga would start on the new moon, with ovulation yoga on the full moon and so on. If teaching pregnant or postpartum students, use your knowledge from your pregnancy and postnatal yoga teacher training or refer to a qualified colleague.

As we are not nutritionists or psychotherapists but are here to support through yoga, we cannot comment on diets or mental health. This is a time to refer to a specialist. But yoga has excellent benefits for our mental and emotional wellbeing and is a great support for our students. It also reflects on how we choose to nourish ourselves through diet if the relationship to food is a challenge. Body-positive and trauma-informed yoga approaches are beneficial in the case of disordered eating or disordered body image.

Whether the reason is *vāta*, *pitta* or *kapha*, we can use an approach to calm the mind and become embodied. This is not about meditation to escape our body and sensations in the body, but rather a way to truly feel what's going on in the body with compassion and without judgement.

Include breathing practices such as diaphragmatic breathing to experience how the body moves with the breath. Heart-womb breath is another embodied practice of resting one hand on the lower abdomen (near the womb space) and the other on the sternum (our energetic heart). Experience the breath rising from womb to (energetic) heart on the inhale and descend on the exhale. Through touch, we can feel the body and the movement of breath. Simply resting the hands over the lower abdomen, perhaps in *shakti* or *yoni mudrā*, is another way to bring awareness to the uterus. As the saying goes: '*prāṇa* flows where attention goes'. And we want *prāṇa* in the reproductive system if we don't ovulate or menstruate.

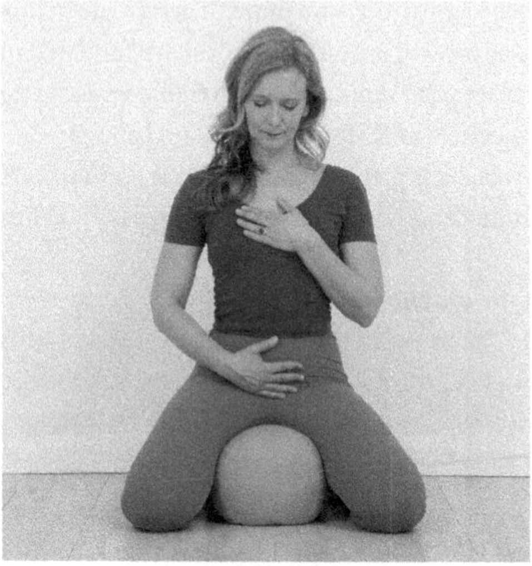

Heart-womb meditation or breathing practice

Most yoga poses can be focused on the pelvis and with pelvic organ awareness. Look at the poses for the (late) luteal phase. All the pelvic rocking, twists, forward bends and backbends stimulate the lower abdomen, bringing circulation and energy to the area. Hip-opening poses such as *kapotāsana* (pigeon pose) also create stimulation and space for the pelvic organs and bring energy to the pelvic bowl. Use the extra stimulation or pressure of the student's own fists or a rolled-up towel/blanket in poses such as *bālāsana* (child's pose) or lunges. These variations are all excellent for amenorrhea.

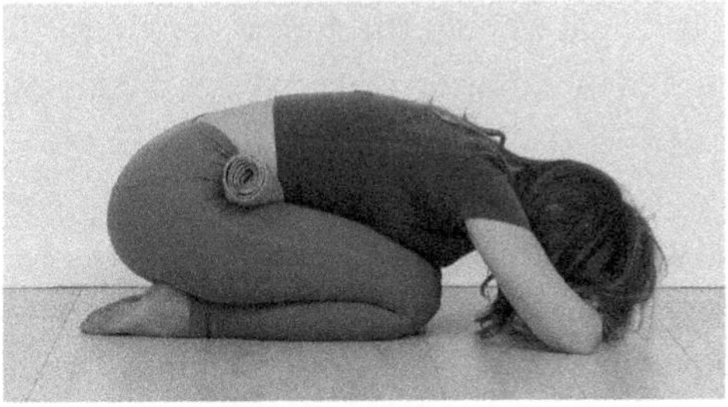

Bālāsana with a rolled-up towel at the lower abdomen

Mālāsana (yogīc squat) is the perfect *apāna vāyu* increasing pose. It is grounding and releases the energy down and out. Squats are a good addition to the yoga sequence with appropriate modification when needed.

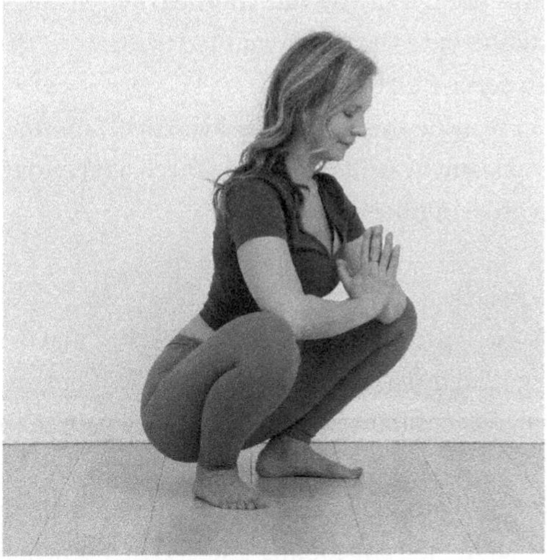

Modify mālāsana by resting the heels on support or sit on a block

Standing poses such as *vīrabhadrāsana* (warrior poses) and *vṛkāsana* (tree pose) are all solid, strong and invoke stability and connection to the earth – being embodied and in our body.

For poses that can create strong sensations such as *kapotāsana* (pigeon pose), lizard pose (deep lunges) or similar poses, encourage experiencing any sensations with a trauma-informed awareness. No judgement, no analysing. No need to go deeper. No need to run away – unless the body tells you to shift out of the pose or it feels unsafe.

If you are a trained yoga *nidra* facilitator this is a beautiful practice to experience the body and different sensations, allowing feelings such as hot and cold, heavy and light without attachment or judgement. Yoga *nidra* is a wonderful practice in mindfulness that can be useful for our students.

Painful ovulation (*mittelschmerz*)

Western perspective

Some people experience pain in the area around one of the ovaries or the lower abdomen when they ovulate. There is no medical term for this but it is sometimes referred to using the German description *mittel* (middle) *schmerz* (pain) as ovulation is generally around the middle of the cycle.

The pain usually only lasts a short time or up to a few hours as ovulation is only a short event. No one knows why it happens. The theory is that when the egg breaks through the ovary wall it releases a bit of fluid which can cause irritation. It could potentially be due to underlying causes such as endometriosis, scar tissue or sexually transmitted diseases irritating the ovaries (National Health Service 2019b).

There is no cure aside from stopping ovulation (and therefore the menstrual cycle) completely by using hormones such as the contraceptive pill. It can be treated with painkillers.

Āyurvedic perspective

When we discussed *Āyurvedic* physiology we learned that ovulation happens when the spark ignited by *pitta* releases an egg. *Pitta* is hot and sharp and *vāta* is the movement. This combination could produce pain in the lower belly or groin. If someone experiences ovulatory pain it could be due to high *pitta doṣa* and the treatment protocol would be to reduce *pitta* in their lifestyle and diet. This means taking it easy, cooling and calming down; no spicy food or alcohol; reducing stress and excess striving or ambition; calming down the ego. Remember that there could also be underlying causes such as scar tissue or endometriosis. If that's the case, always look at the root cause.

Yoga practices for painful ovulation

If your client tends to experience increased *pitta* look at cooling and calming down through yoga, breathing and meditation, especially around ovulation. Even though the follicular phase is great to create strength, power and a little heat, be mindful that any *pitta* students shouldn't push themselves too far. Create softness, calmness and coolness in their practice. It is always better to prevent something than having to navigate the discomfort once it's manifest.

Sheetali (cooling) breath is appropriate as a general practice but also during ovulatory pain. *Brāmari prāṇayāma* (bumblebee) is another breathing practice to calm down anger and irritation in the mind. *Nāḍīśodhana* (alternate nostril breathing) is a beautiful balancing practice at any time. Focus on opening the space around the lower abdomen with *setubandhāsana* (bridge pose) and *suptabaddhakoṇāsana* (reclined goddess/cobbler's pose).

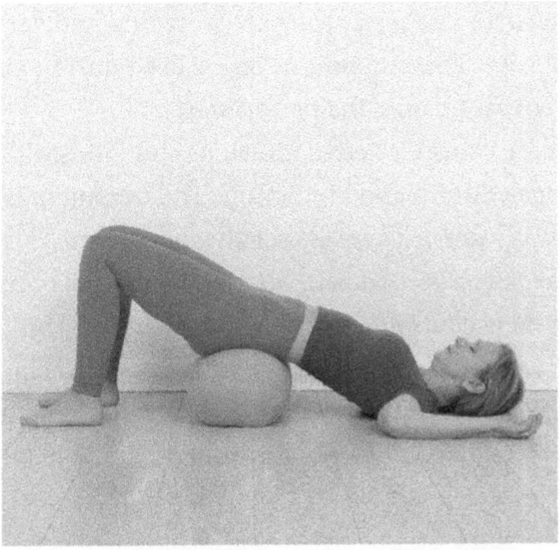

Setubandhāsana variation with a bolster under the pelvis

Painful periods (dysmenorrhea) and cramps

Western perspective

Cramps causing painful periods are fairly common. The uterus, or womb, is the strongest muscle in the human body. It expels the menstrual fluid (endometrial lining and blood) through contractions, just like the uterus expels the baby or babies and placenta during childbirth through uterine contractions. The uterus has to be strong. These contractions are what we experience as menstrual cramps or painful periods. But it should not be so painful or create extreme cramps that you double over in agony.

The contractions are caused by prostaglandins which increase in the body at the beginning of the menstrual phase. These hormone-like substances occur naturally as part of the healing process when we have an injury or infection as well as during our period. Although necessary for the menstrual cycle, high levels of prostaglandins can cause inflammation, swelling, menstrual pain and cramps. They can also seep out to other tissues and cause issues such as lower backache and nausea.

Āyurvedic perspective

Vāta is often the culprit of pain. *Vāta* is also movement, which is what cramps and contractions are. The qualities of *vāta doṣa* are cold, dry, irregularity, fast and rough. With excess *vāta*, we try to reduce *vāta* qualities and encourage the opposites. This can be warming herbal teas, slowing down, a hot water bottle and relaxed calming yoga poses. Castor oil packs are often recommended in *vāta*-related menstrual issues as they are warming and very oily, breaking up any dried up *vāta*. These should never be used during menstruation but rather as a preventative before the period starts.

In *Āyurveda*, we consider herbal infusions and foods with warming qualities such as ginger, cumin and cinnamon. The treatment is to balance and create a free flow of *vāta* or *vāyu*, especially *apāna vāyu*.

Although we generally associate *vāta* with pain, the other *doṣas* can also manifest as painful periods. *Pitta* pain is mostly hot and inflamed and needs a more cooling and soothing approach which could include a cool rather than a hot compress. *Kapha*-dominant people experience a more dull and heavy discomfort. *Kapha* pain needs warmth and some movement to release stagnation.

Yoga practices for menstrual pain and cramps

Backbends seem to be a common theme for many of the scientific studies on *yogāsana* and menstrual pain (Satyanand *et al.* 2014; Rakhshaee 2011). These include *setubandhāsana* (bridge pose), *matsyandrāsana* (lord of the fishes), *bhujangāsana* (cobra pose) and *dhanurāsana* (wheel). Evidence shows that abdominal stretching is effective in decreasing pain during menstruation (Rejeki *et al.* 2021; Bustan, Seweng & Ernawati 2018). One study (Motahari-Tabari, Shirvani & Alipour 2017, p.47) shows that 'Stretching exercises were as effective as mefenamic acid in the treatment of primary dysmenorrhea' (mefenamic acid is a prescription drug for period pain). The exercises weren't performed during menstruation but three times a week through the month and it was suggested that 'the effect of exercise on relieving menstruation pain increases over time'.

We can include these poses throughout the menstrual cycle as a preventative to open and create space in the lower abdomen so that *vāta doṣa*, and *apāna vāyu*, can flow in its natural direction.

Supported restorative or *yin*-style yoga poses work well. These are another opportunity to soothe the body, the nervous system and *vāta doṣa*, so we can breathe calmly. This can help ease the contractions and tensions of the body (and mind) that may exacerbate the intense cramping.

Try a supported *setubandhāsana* (bridge pose) with a bolster or yoga blocks under the pelvis and *suptabaddhakoṇāsana* (reclined Goddess/cobbler's pose) with support under the thighs or perhaps reclining over a bolster as well. Both these poses create space and openness to release tension around the pelvis and lower abdomen. According to some research, 'abdominal stretching exercise can be an alternative choice of management of dysmenorrhea' (Rosyida *et al.* 2017).

Balāsana (child's pose) is perhaps a natural position for the body to take when in pain. Folding over a bolster offers a bit more space and comfort.

Personally, I find sitting cross-legged and gently rocking while using a soft *ujjâyî prāṇayāma* or humming (*Brāmari prāṇayāma*) are meditative ways to ease these strong sensations.

In any of the poses, the focus is to slow down the breath to calm both body and mind, essentially soothing the excessive movement of *vāta doṣa*.

Yoga *nidra* is also yoga. We don't always have to focus on *āsana*. One study (Monika *et al.* 2012, p.166) suggests 'that after yoga nidra practice patients relieved from painful cramps, heavy bleeding and irregular periods'. That's a pretty powerful message of the importance of taking time to rest.

Pelvic pain

Western perspective

A client may present with a diagnosis of pelvic pain. This is a description covering many different symptoms and issues so we need to ask more questions. Chronic pelvic pain can be defined as non-cyclical pain lasting six months or more affecting the pelvis, anterior abdominal wall, lower back, or buttocks that is serious enough to affect one's quality of life and needing medical care (Broderick, Kennedy & Zondervan 2013).

Generally, pelvic pain is a pain in the pelvis or lower abdomen. It can be a result of some of the complaints discussed here such as endometriosis, cysts and fibroids. It can also be a digestive issue such as constipation, irritable bowel syndrome and inflammatory bowel disease, or due to appendicitis, peritonitis and cystitis or urinary tract infection. The pain can be related to pelvic inflammatory disease, caused by bacteria in the reproductive system. This bacteria is sometimes due to sexually transmitted diseases, which can be another cause of pelvic pain.

Prolapse, hernia and nerve pain are other reasons for pelvic pain. Pelvic girdle pain includes sacroiliac joint pain, pubis symphysis dysfunction and pain in the joints of the pelvic bowl. This is something we often hear about during pregnancy or postpartum but everybody can experience pelvic girdle pain.

Like all muscles, the pelvic floor muscles can become tight, strained and have tension causing pelvic pain.

It's not just physical causes that manifest as pelvic pain. The pain can be due to trauma (which could be physical or emotional) as well as general stress and anxiety.

There are many potential causes of pelvic pain. The symptoms relevant to menstrual and cyclic health are discussed separately – that is the focus of this book. However, everything is related. I believe that tightness and imbalance of the pelvic floor muscles, as well as the alignment of the pelvic area in general, can cause issues around the uterus and ovaries via the fascia and ligaments, which may result in menstrual complaints. Practising yoga, we have an incredible opportunity to connect with this area to create balance. The pelvis and pelvic floor is something I am passionate about. We need to get educated – as do our students. It's beyond the scope of this book but it is something I discuss in my dedicated pelvis and pelvic floor immersion, the Sacred Pelvis, on my website (https://yogaembodiedonline.com).

Āyurvedic perspective

As there are so many symptoms, please refer to the complaints related to the menstrual cycle that we cover in this chapter, whether it is endometriosis, polycystic ovary syndrome or another symptom. However, I do want to share a couple of thoughts on the pelvis and pelvic pain in general.

The pelvis is the seat, or home, of *vāta doṣa*, specifically *apāna vāyu*. Most issues in this area will relate to *vāta* and *apāna vāyu*. Maybe there is too much *vāta* or *apāna* and not enough support and structure. Maybe *vāta* moves in the wrong direction. *Vāta* is about mobility and can 'push' the other *doṣas*. This means either *pitta* or *kapha* or both can be involved, for example by accumulating or being pushed into other tissues.

From both a Western and *Āyurvedic* perspective, digestion is another reason for pelvic complaints and *Āyurveda* has a great belief that digestion is one of the pillars of health. This is a subject we can't go into here but there are plenty of resources on good digestive health and it is something I explain in my Detox & Rejuvenate online course (and yes, I include the importance of *rasāyana*, or rejuvenation, too).

Pain in the pelvis can be psychological and emotional. From an *Āyurvedic* and yoga perspective, this makes sense. *Vāta* is our nervous system. Any trauma and stress will affect *vāta* and the nervous system. Another of *vāta*'s qualities is pain. If there is a lot of pain there is often *vāta*.

From a more modern psychological yoga perspective, the root, *mūlādhāra*, and the sacral, *svādhiṣṭhāna*, *cakras* are situated in the pelvis. These are said to relate to safety, security, family, network, culture, sexuality and creative expression. Anything that feels as if it threatens our safety, security and truth might manifest physically in the areas of those *cakras*. This also relates to our nervous system (*vāta*) and how we tighten the respiratory and pelvic diaphragm (pelvic floor) during anxiety and stress, or through the fight, flight or freeze response, which in turn can affect the rest of the pelvic bowl and pelvic organs.

Yoga practices for pelvic pain

If there is a specific complaint, look at the reference for that particular issue. From an *Āyurvedic* perspective, we can explore the relationship between the seat of *vāta* and *apāna*, the *cakras* and the nervous system.

There is limited research into yoga for pelvic pain but one systematic review (Russell *et al.* 2019, p.153) concludes that there is 'moderate evidence to support the use of yoga to improve pain and psychological and emotional QOL (quality of life) domains in women with CPP (chronic pelvic pain)'.

Another study (Gonçalves *et al.* 2016, p.977) referring to endometriosis reports how, 'women said they had identified a relationship between pain management and breathing techniques (*prāṇayāma*) learned in yoga and that breathing increased their ability to be introspective, which relieved pain'. In yoga classes, we connect with the breath and the connection between body, breath and mind. It can be an immensely powerful way to navigate through issues such as pelvic pain.

As much as many yoga teachers have been indoctrinated to engage the *mūlabandha* as a way to connect to and strengthen the pelvic floor, we also need to be aware that a too tight pelvic floor can lead to pelvic pain, incontinence and general discomfort, as can any other hypertonic or tense muscles. We need to relax the pelvic floor. Encouraging proper diaphragmatic breathing will allow the pelvic floor to move with the breath. This way we can use breath as a way to manage pain.

Add in yoga poses to help release tension in general and specifically around the pelvis and pelvic floor. Include *upaviṣṭakoṇāsana* (wide-legged seated pose), *malāsana* (squat) variations, and *adhomukhaśvānāsana* (downward-facing dog), with emphasis on widening the sitting bones. Hip-opening poses such as *kapotāsana* (pigeon pose) or fire log pose/double pigeon both stretch the outer hips and glutes to ease the muscles of the pelvis. *Viparīta karaṇī* (legs-up-the-wall) or resting the lower legs on a chair while lying on the floor with knees bent are both excellent ways to relax the pelvic area, hips and the mind. One of the techniques I mentioned to navigate pain during the menstrual phase was to sit cross-legged and gently rock forwards and backwards using a meditative *ujjayi prāṇayāma*. This could also be useful here.

Premenstrual syndrome (PMS) and premenstrual dysphoric disorder (PMDD)

Western perspective

Premenstrual syndrome is the name for all the various symptoms one can experience just before menstruation. These include mood swings, anxiety, irritability, fatigue, feeling emotional, feeling bloated, having tender breasts, greasy hair and skin, headaches and changes in appetite and libido.

Premenstrual dysphoric disorder is when the symptoms are extremely severe. It's when feeling a bit emotional or low becomes being depressed, having panic attacks or feeling suicidal. It's when craving chocolate becomes extreme binge eating, or when feeling uncomfortable in body or mind becomes painful.

The causes of either are not known (National Health Service 2021c). But it is thought to be due to the changes in hormones affecting us at this time in the cycle. For people with PMDD there seems to be a correlation with a specific sensitivity to the hormonal changes.

The Western approach is to stop the cycle altogether by prescribing hormones such as the contraceptive pill. For some symptoms, cognitive behavioural therapy can be prescribed, or potentially antidepressants.

If someone has PMDD they will need professional support. Yoga can be complementary to that.

Āyurvedic perspective

The symptoms here are all different expressions of *doṣic* imbalances highlighted at the time before the menstrual phase. This is when the strong sharp focused *pitta* can push symptoms to the surface.

Let's look at the individual *doṣas* and how they might manifest during the premenstrual phase:

> *Vāta*: anxiety, fear, insomnia and mood swings; bloating and wind; lower back and leg ache and pain in the lower abdomen.
>
> *Pitta*: irritability and anger; headaches and migraines; hot and inflamed skin including acne; tender swollen breasts; soft bowel movements.
>
> *Kapha*: feeling low, emotional, tearful; sleepy and sluggish; feeling swollen, bloated and puffy with water retention; swollen breasts.

We have already looked at acne, fatigue and water retention. We always look at the individual and focus on reducing and pacifying the vitiated *doṣa*, perhaps bringing in some of the opposite qualities as well. We must remember that we don't just deal with the symptoms when they manifest as PMS but throughout the cycle. *Āyurveda* is a lifestyle, not just a quick pill to suppress a symptom.

Yoga practices for PMS

Because each symptom has a different cause, we will look at the cause, not just the symptom. If someone has high *vāta* it is not just during their premenstrual phase, it is a part of their personality or lifestyle. Even throughout their monthly yoga programme, we need to be aware we don't vitiate their *vāta* but encourage its reduction. The same goes for *pitta* and *kapha*. We are pacifying whatever has been aggravated by reducing those qualities in life and in the yoga practice.

You can go back to Chapter 3 and the introduction to *Āyurveda* where we mentioned what the qualities of the different *doṣas* are and how to reduce them in general. Here is a quick reminder:

Vāta: Keep warm, slow and steady. Get grounded. Be in the body, not the mind. Consider the menstrual yoga practice for inspiration and encourage what we explored in Chapter 13 on rest.

Pitta: Stay cool and calm by slowing down the practice and reducing any form of competitiveness and ego. Burned-out *pittas* need to get permission to stop or slow down and practise what we discussed in Chapter 13 on the importance of rest. Both the luteal and menstrual phase inspired yoga are balancing for *pitta*. Introduce the philosophy and spiritual practice of yoga and the concept of *sattva*.

Kapha: *Kapha* people need to breathe fully and exercise their lungs with more dynamic practices. This also includes their *āsana* practice, where movement is key. This *doṣa* might want to rest and slow down but is the one *doṣa* where activity is encouraged, and the follicular phase yoga is perfect for *kapha*.

Polycystic ovary syndrome (PCOS)

Western perspective

There is no definite answer to why some people develop polycystic ovary syndrome. It is a rather complex set of symptoms that involves metabolism, hormones and the reproductive system.

The National Health and Medical Research Council's (2018) PCOS guidelines explain that 'Women with PCOS present with diverse features including psychological (anxiety, depression, body image), reproductive (irregular menstrual cycles, hirsutism, infertility and pregnancy complications) and metabolic features (insulin resistance (IR), metabolic syndrome, prediabetes, type 2 diabetes (DM2) and cardiovascular risk factors).' Although it is inconclusive, it seems to be an issue around lack of ovulation which leads to lack of menstruation. It is important to know that we can all have cysts on the ovaries which can come and go. This does not necessarily mean we have PCOS or that we are even aware of it.

With its numerous symptoms, PCOS is challenging for setting a treatment protocol, let alone understanding the underlying cause. Hormones seem to be the main factor, whether it is insulin resistance, higher levels of testosterone or luteinizing hormone, or lower levels of sex hormone-binding globulin.

Hormonal therapy such as the pill or the coil (intrauterine device) is sometimes offered, which is contraception affecting the natural menstrual and ovulatory cycle.

Āyurvedic perspective

Imbalanced *vāta* or *apāna vāyu* have likely caused an obstruction in the pelvis leading *kapha* as well as *pitta* to accumulate and create the cysts (Dayani Siriwardene *et al.* 2010).

Vāta's seat is the pelvis. *Kapha* is building and accumulating and *pitta* is related to blood, *rakta dhātu*, and how we view hormones in Western medicine.

As always, we look at the whole picture. Diet is of great importance in *Āyurveda* when it comes to our general health and wellbeing. This is especially important in PCOS where some people experience weight gain and have issues around insulin (prediabetes). However, in *Āyurveda* this is also about the concept of *āma* or how well we digest, metabolize and release what we eat. Any *āma* can create build-up and manifest as illness such as PCOS. This does not mean we, as yoga teachers, offer diet advice or detox suggestions. In *Āyurveda*, this would be done by an *Āyurvedic* doctor or practitioner following the principles of *pañchakarma*, a very specific cleansing programme.

Yoga practices for PCOS

In the complexity of the various symptoms and potentially different causes of PCOS, we can support our students depending on how they feel at the time we see them.

If the student is mainly anxious, we can create yoga to regulate and soothe the nervous system. If they happen to be overweight and want support with fitness, we can practise *yogāsana* for physical exercise, yet also support body positivity and the nervous system, embracing yoga's holistic approach. If fertility and trying to conceive is the main objective, we can use the guidance we discussed under fertility.

Some of the symptoms of PCOS include very irregular or absent periods. But it is not just a lack of periods, it could also be that there is no ovulation. We look at our students as individuals and adjust accordingly rather than apply the cyclical phase yoga practices, as they may not experience ovulation or menstruation. If this is the case, we can work with the moon and use yoga according to the phases of the moon. Practise menstrual yoga at the new moon and ovulation yoga around the full moon. Encourage the abundance, fertility (not necessarily to procreate but as a sign of health), juiciness and sensuality of the full moon. Even if the student does not ovulate, we can welcome and encourage that same energy.

To break up any vitiated or obstructed *kapha doṣa* we need dynamic movement and breathing such as *sūryanamaskāra* (sun salutations) and a steady breath-connected *vinyāsa* flow. Include plenty of twists to stimulate circulation around the intestines, digestive system and lower abdomen where the pelvic organs reside. Add in the compression of the lower abdomen as we mentioned in yoga for the follicular phase.

To calm down *vāta* or any anxiety include breathing practices for balance, such as *nāḍīśōdhana* (alternate nostril breathing). Enjoy hip-opening poses including *kapotāsana* (pigeon pose), *mālāsana* (squat variations), *suptabaddhakoṇāsana* (reclined Goddess or cobbler's pose) as well as supported *setubandhāsana* (bridge pose). Include the *vāta*-reducing *pawanmukasana* (wind-releasing exercises) for digestion (which is great for a sluggish *kapha doṣa* too).

Several research papers (Patel *et al.* 2020; Vanitha *et al.* 2018; Nidhi *et al.* 2012) show that yoga and yoga *nidra* helps to improve the quality of life in individuals with PCOS. In one paper, *sūryanamaskāra* (sun salutations), *ardhāmatsyendrāsana* (half lord of the fishes pose), *bharadvajāsana* (seated spinal twist), *baddhakonāsana* (cobbler's/butterfly pose), *suptabaddhakonāsana* (reclining butterfly pose), *ushtrāsana* (camel pose) and *sarvangāsana* (shoulderstand) were some of the recommended poses. They also recommended *prāṇayāma* including *kapālabhāti* (cleansing breath), *ujjâyî* (ocean sound breath) and *anuloma viloma* (alternate nostril breathing) (Kadam *et al.* 2014).

Yoga can also be beneficial for people with PCOS undergoing fertility treatment with the additional stress and anxiety that may bring (Mohseni *et al.* 2021).

CHAPTER 15

Hormone Therapy, Hormonal Birth Control and the Pill

This whole book is about the natural phases of menstruation, the follicular phase, ovulation and the luteal phase. However, many of our students may not actually menstruate (although they may think they are) or indeed ovulate. This includes students on the pill or other hormonal contraception.

Your students may be on hormonal contraception (such as the pill) because they use it as birth control. However, if you have read through the chapter on common complaints you now know that many people are prescribed hormonal contraception as a way to alleviate the presented symptoms, not to prevent pregnancy. Because hormonal contraception can stop ovulation and menstruation, many of the challenges associated with the cycle may be alleviated. However, it also stops the natural hormonal and *doṣic* fluctuations and the benefits that come with the different phases of the menstrual cycle. In *Āyurveda*, we look at things slightly differently. We explore potential imbalances that have caused the complaints and aim to create balance again. This includes the *Āyurvedic* principles you are learning about and the yoga you already know and are expanding on.

So, what is hormonal contraception and hormone therapy?

Combined pill

This is the regular pill that has synthetic variations of oestrogen (estradiol) and progesterone. These are not the same as what we produce naturally in the body. The pill shuts down the natural ovulatory phase, meaning you neither ovulate nor menstruate. Any breakthrough bleed experienced is a response to the drug (or rather drug withdrawal, as the bleeding is in the non-drug phase), not regular natural menstruation.

Progestogen-only pill (POP), mini pill

This pill has no oestrogen but a progestin. The mini pill works by affecting the mucus in the cervix to stop sperm from entering the uterus. According to Patient.info (Willacy 2021), 'POPs also have some effect on the ovary. Your ovaries do not release an egg (ovulate) as often when you take the POP. The newer type of POP containing desogestrel stops ovulation most of the time. Stopping ovulation is the main way these newer pills work.' Again, this is a drug that stops the natural phases of the cycle.

Implant

This is a bit like the progestogen-only pill except that it is implanted into the upper arm. It works by thickening the mucus at the cervix to prevent the sperm from entering the uterus. It also prevents ovulation, meaning you do not have a menstrual or ovulatory cycle.

The patch

The patch is very similar to the combined pill except that the hormones enter the body through the skin rather than through oral administration. With oestrogen (estradiol) and a progesterone-like hormone, it prevents a natural cycle of ovulation and menstruation.

The vaginal ring

This is like the combined pill with both estradiol and a progestin suppressing ovulation and therefore the cycle.

Intrauterine system (IUS)

The coil releases progestogen, which thickens the cervical mucus. This makes it more challenging for sperm to move through the cervix into the uterus. It also thins the lining of the womb so an egg is less likely to be able to implant itself. For some people, the IUS prevents ovulation as well.

Copper intrauterine device (IUD)

I am mentioning the IUD to compare it with the hormonal IUS. This coil does not contain any hormones and is made from copper and plastic. It works by impairing sperm motility and embryo plantation simply by being made of copper and being in the uterus. There is still a cycle but periods can become heavier using the copper IUD.

Contraceptive injection

The contraceptive injection releases progestogen, which thickens the cervical mucus. This makes it more challenging for sperm to move through the cervix into the uterus. It also thins the lining of the womb so an egg is less likely to be able to implant.

Recap of hormonal contraception

In these hormonal methods of contraception, the natural cycle is suppressed. Often there is no bleed even if there might be ovulation (in case of contraceptive injection, for example). They can still give irregular, heavy or very light bleeds (which are not menstruation), sometimes no bleeding at all.

Although artificial hormones may be the best option for some, it is worth noting that they do disrupt the natural hormones completely and there is no natural cycle. The artificial hormones do not act in the same way. There are other options for contraception such as barrier methods (condoms, cap, diaphragm) and the natural fertility method.

Hormone replacement therapy (HRT)

This is sometimes prescribed during the perimenopause and postmenopause. It can also be offered after a hysterectomy where the ovaries have been removed.

HRT contains an oestrogen-like hormone to 'replace' the oestrogen the ovaries would produce during regular cyclic living (before the perimenopause) and is usually combined with a progestogen hormone. In the case of a hysterectomy, where there are no longer any ovaries to produce oestrogen, an oestrogen-only hormone replacement may be prescribed.

Again, any bleeding is not a period and there is no longer any ovulation.

Breast cancer and hormone therapy

Some breast cancers are stimulated by oestrogen or progesterone. Treatment can include using hormone therapy to lower these stimulants either before or after chemotherapy and potential surgery. Hormone therapy is closely monitored with the client's consultant.

However, it means that some of our students with, or recovering from, breast cancer may not have a menstrual cycle. If they have a sense of shifts and phases in their body or energy, they can listen to their body wisdom or follow the moon cycles.

Cyclic living with no menstruation or ovulation

It is not our place to educate on contraception, hormones or HRT. We can encourage our students to educate themselves, learn about their bodies and make informed choices.

When our students don't have an actual cycle, yet want to explore this approach to yoga and as a way of living, they can:

- work with their induced hormonal cycle. If they are on the pill and have regular breakthrough bleeds, they can still work with the phases
- work with the moon phases if there is no cyclic phases or signs of breakthrough bleeding
- be intuitive and listen to their own body wisdom.

Body wisdom is what yoga and *Āyurveda* are about. Is *vāta* vitiated today? Then practise a routine to calm *vāta* such as the menstrual phase yoga, even if there is no menstruation. Do they feel strong and have good stamina although feeling a little sluggish, like *kapha*? Then be creative with the follicular or ovulation phase yoga. Is there sharpness and motivation with strong yet regular *pitta*? Then enjoy the early luteal yoga sequencing.

In the end, it is about finding what works for the individual – not the ego, but the body, mind, emotions and energy.

CHAPTER 16

Perimenopause Leading to Change

Transitioning beyond the menstrual cycle

Western perspective

Let's first define the menopause. The menopause is the day you haven't had a period for one whole year. That's it – one day. This may be confusing as many people, including health professionals, talk about the menopause and menopausal symptoms as years of transitioning in our forties and fifties. This time of transition is in fact the perimenopause. Peri means 'around' and perimenopause refers to the time leading up to the menopause. This is usually a transition taking about seven years but could be longer or shorter. The average age for the menopause in the UK is 51 (National Health Service 2018).

The time after the menopause is sometimes referred to as the postmenopause. At this time, most symptoms from the transition into the menopause (perimenopause) should settle (although it can take longer for some individuals) and it's a transition into a new state of hormonal balance.

We discussed the perimenopause in Chapter 9 and I am including this short chapter because there is still a menstrual cycle and there is still ovulation although it can be more irregular and sometimes be missing altogether for a while. We are not going into details about what happens in the perimenopause or postmenopause because this stage of life truly deserves a book on its own.

Here is a brief overview of what may be experienced in the perimenopause. Just like menarche, the time we get our first period, hormones are fluctuating and changing. And just like menarche, the periods can get heavy, irregular and painful, or perhaps super light and easy. Sometimes there is no ovulation. Sometimes we miss a period. Perhaps the cycle shortens. There might be weight gain, mood swings, brain fog, hot flushes and night sweats. Some people experience more symptoms and find the transition extremely challenging. Others have hardly any discomfort, but rather they feel empowered with the hormonal shifts.

Why does this happen? The hormones are changing. This is one reason why hormonal tests aren't reliable as a way of diagnosing the perimenopause. Oestrogen can increase dramatically and then suddenly crash. We know of oestrogen as a hormone that makes us feel more at ease and stronger mentally and physically. It is no wonder many people experience extreme mood swings during this time. Progesterone is also slowly declining. This is the calming and soothing hormone.

Āyurvedic perspective

From an *Āyurvedic* perspective, any change relates to *vāta doṣa*. The perimenopause is a sudden change from decades of menstrual cycles to very irregular (another *vāta* quality) cycles and finally no cycle at all.

Of course, the other *doṣas* are involved too. Hormones are often associated with *pitta*, and *vāta* is certainly influencing the hormones affecting *pitta doṣa*. Most of us also continue with the *pitta* mindset of doing, ambition and accomplishment during the perimenopause, which will show up as aggravated *pitta* symptoms at this time. We will look at those in a moment.

You may remember how in *Āyurveda* everything has different stages. For example, childhood is affected by *kapha doṣa* with its qualities of building up, growth and strength. *Pitta doṣa* is adulthood with its fire to create, and to have the ambition to work and make a living. As we get older, we need less. We come into the *vāta* stage of air and space. We don't need to build up and grow the same way as we did as children. And we don't need the same fire to work and accomplish things as we did in mid-life. Now we can let go and start to focus on the spiritual path. This is the positive side of the lightness of *vāta doṣa*. We can pursue our inner work, reflection and insight, connecting to the wisdom we have gathered through the years.

If any of the *doṣas* are imbalanced they can manifest as typical perimenopause characteristics:

Vāta: insomnia and anxiety; potential for bone loss leading to osteopenia and osteoporosis; dryness, including drier skin, vaginal dryness and vaginal atrophy; constipation and bloating.

Pitta: excess heat in the body leads to irritation and inflammation of the skin but also anger and irritability; severe mood swings; night sweats and hot flushes; heavier periods.

Kapha: feeling low, depressed and unmotivated; weight gain and fluid retention; feeling slow and experiencing sluggish digestion.

Yoga practices at perimenopause

Because everybody is different, there is no one solution or one yoga sequence that is perfect for the perimenopause. We evaluate the individual. We look at the way we live, our lifestyle and how we feel rather than masking a problem. Prevention is always better than trying to find a solution once a symptom has occurred.

In *Āyurveda*, we know perimenopause is a transition to the *vāta* stage of being. So we offer *vāta*-balancing support. This includes the importance of rest and increasing *ojas*, as we discussed in Chapter 13 on rest. These solutions can also help to cool down excess *pitta doṣa*.

As we live in a culture where the *pitta* characteristics of being busy, ambitious and 'doing' all the time are appreciated and celebrated, we need to create more balance in our lifestyle. We need to slow down, take time to be. Although we do want some stamina, we don't want to overheat. Even food and beverages that are heating, such as alcohol and spicy foods, can be reduced. Digestion and movement are important so we don't slumber into a lethargic and heavy excessive *kapha* or *tāmasic* state.

It is all about balance.

When a student is in the perimenopause, discuss any general complaints to create a yoga programme for prevention, and work with the student once symptoms are present. If your student currently experiences heavy periods, look at the section on heavy periods in Chapter 14. Have a look at the section on PMS for emotional balance. Always include aspects from Chapter 13 on the importance of rest.

Final Reflections

This book is very special to me. It's an expression of my passions; my love for yoga and my deep respect for the wisdom of *Āyurveda*. Both have impacted my life immensely. It is also an appreciation of the wise women who came before, who shared the wisdom, power and sacredness of the menstrual cycle and the Feminine. This is wisdom that was lost through time and is now slowly starting to be rediscovered.

On *Āyurveda*

In a way, *Āyurveda* is pretty simple. Once you appreciate the five great elements and the three *doṣas* you can apply them to everything: your yoga, diet and how you move through the day, the seasons, the year and life cycles. So, if the information in this book sometimes feels overwhelming, go back to the basics. If your client has excess *pitta doṣa*, reduce heating practices and favour a more cooling and calming approach. With increased *kapha doṣa*, embrace movement and lightness rather than stagnant and heavy qualities in your teaching. A vitiated *vata* personality needs to get grounded and calm the mind rather than having too much lightness and spaciousness. It is the same with the external environment; your teachings will change depending on whether it is a hot, sunny day or a cold, wet winter morning. And that's how you apply the *Āyurvedic* principles to the menstrual cycle too.

Āyurveda is also very complex. If you are an *Āyurvedic* practitioner, this book presents a very simplified approach to *Āyurveda* and yoga. There is much more information on physiology and diagnostics when we look at the menstrual cycle and the individual person from an *Āyurveda* perspective, but perhaps this book has inspired you to learn more.

I hope I have found the balance of offering enough understanding and appreciation of *Āyurveda* without it being overwhelming, yet not over simplifying such a vast and sometimes complex system.

On the menstrual cycle

The changing phases of the inner and outer lunar cycles are incredible. The more I research, explore and read the more fascinated I get. The most powerful teachings are through my embodied experience of the menstrual cycle. But whether you menstruate or not, I invite you to honour these changing cycles, to appreciate the changing rhythms of the physical body and energetic being through the menstrual cycle. Allow the menstrual cycle to become a guide in our lives and pay attention to Mother Nature. Menstruation and the cycle are powerful.

On embodying and teaching

This book is for education, information and inspiration. It's the practical application and embodied experience that matter.

Now it is up to you to digest and assimilate this information so it can inform and enhance how you teach and share your yoga.

Enjoy the journey.

Acknowledgements

There are so many people who, in their own way, have been a part of this journey – even if not very obvious. Thank you.

Thank you to all my yoga teachers and *Āyurveda* teachers. To my teacher Shiva Rea, who shares yoga, *Āyurveda* and feminine flow. I have many *Āyurvedic* teachers and doctors in my life. All have inspired me and have been – and still are – an important part of my journey. Thank you, Dr Mathew, for supporting me through my menstrual cycles, reminding me of the 'white coat syndrome' when I presented with many of the issues I share in this book, and thank you for writing the foreword. Gratitude to Dr Robert Svoboda and my *Āyurveda* teachers at Middlesex University, SDM College of Ayurveda and Hospital, AVP Hospital and KLE University.

As is often said, much gratitude to all my teachers and my teachers' teachers, the great sages of *Āyurveda* and yoga.

The practical writing and editing couldn't have been done without two incredible people: Mel Cole, who not only offered suggestions and edits but also created all the illustrations, and Eana Vagjiani – without her edits, encouragement, optimism and friendship this book wouldn't be the same. Thank you. I also want to thank friend, obstetrician and gynaecologist Dr Monalisa Neogi for all our pelvic health conversations. I am grateful to Pete Muller, who did all the photos of me for the book and to Salt Water Studio for providing the beautiful yoga space. Gratitude to the team at Singing Dragon for being supportive of this book.

Writing has always been something I enjoyed as a creative process, even as a child, late at night when I couldn't sleep. Thank you to my parents for encouraging my creativity (*Tak mor*).

The process of writing this book has been incredible – and not always easy. Thank you to my husband Dan for being there, and affirming I could do this; to Mama Ocean and my mermates for keeping me cool and calm.

A huge thank you to all the people who have come to my classes, workshops, talks, training courses and consultations, and have shared their questions and helped form the offerings I provide, including this book. You are my teachers, I learn from you and with you.

I bow to the Great Mother, the Goddess herself, *Śakti*.

To the God of *Āyurveda, Dhanvantari*.

Oṃ Dhaṃ Dhanvantaraye Namaḥ.

In gratitude. Thank you.

Anja

Glossary

Abhyanga: oil massage of the body either by one self or by an *Āyurvedic* therapist/practitioner.
Agni: fire, including the element of fire and the digestive fire.
Ākāśa: the element of space or ether.
Āma: undigested material or toxins.
Āpa: the element of water.
Apāna vāyu: the downward moving energy of *vāyu* or *vāta.*
Ārtava dhātu: the blood tissue.
Āsana: pose or seat referring to modern yoga postures.
Aṣṭāṅga-hṛdayam: one of the classical *Āyurvedic* texts.
Aṣṭāṅga Vinyāsa yoga: referring the physical *āsana* practice as guided by Pattabhi Jois.
Āyurveda: the science of life and the traditional Indian medical system.
Bandhas: locks or seals.
Bhūmī: the element of earth also called *pṛthvī.*
Cakra: literally a wheel referring to subtle centres in our energetic being. The most commonly known *cakras* are: the root, *mūlādhāra* at the base of the spine, the perineum or the cervix in female anatomy depending on the source. The sacral *cakra*, *svādhiṣṭhāna* behind the pubic bones towards the spine or sacrum. The navel centre, *maṇipūra cakra*. The heart area is called *anāhata.* The throat is *viśuddhi cakra*. The third eye centre is *ājñā cakra*. The *sahasrāra cakra* is the crown of the head and it's debatable if this is even an actual *cakra* or a different energetic centre.
Caraka-saṃhitā: one of the classical *Āyurvedic* texts.
Dhātus: tissues the body is made of, in *Āyurvedic* physiology.
Doṣa/doṣic: literally a fault but meaning the qualities of the five elements in specific combinations. Part of our constitution.
Follicular phase: the time between menstruation and ovulation. In medical textbooks, the early follicular phase includes menstruation.
Guṇas: mean qualities. In yoga, we often refer to the three *guṇas* of the mind: *sattva*, *rajas* and *tamas.*
Haṭha yoga: a specific brand of yoga that includes *āsana.*

Jala: the element of water.

Kapha doṣa: the qualities of the water and earth elements.

Karmendriya: the five organs or means of action: speech, hands, feet, excretion and reproduction.

Kegels: pelvic floor exercises named after the American gynaecologist Arnold Henry Kegel. However, the yoga tradition has always acknowledged pelvic awareness including *mūlabandha* (perineal/pelvic floor/cervical lock), *awshwini* (the anal sphincter engagement) and *sahajolī mudra* (urinary tract area support). I prefer using the word pelvic floor awareness to explore the engagement and release of the pelvic floor muscles rather than Kegel exercises.

Kuṇḍalinī Śakti: literally meaning coiled energy. An energy (*Śakti*) at the base of the spine at the *mūlādhāra cakra* which may rise with energic or spiritual advancement.

Kuṇḍalinī yoga: awareness of *kuṇḍalinī Śakti* and the advancement of spiritual awakening. One modern interpretation was made famous by Yogi Bhajan, an Indian teacher, who brought this practice to the United States and the West. His teachings include energetic movement meditations to raise *kuṇḍalinī Śakti*, which are rather different from most modern yoga classes. There are other interpretations of *kuṇḍalinī* yoga.

Luteal phase: the time between ovulation and menstruation.

Menstruation (in some texts this is also referred to as the early follicular phase): the period or bleed. The time from the first day of bleeding until the bleed is finished.

Mīmāṃsa: one of the *Ṣaḍ-Darśana*, spiritual philosophies, which also include *Sāṅkhya*, *Nyāya*, *Vaiśeṣika*, *Yoga* and *Vedānta*.

Menopause: the day when one hasn't had a period for a whole year.

Mudrā: hand gesture but can also refer to other energetic movements or gestures.

Mūlabandha: the root lock or seal at the base of the spine, perineum or cervix.

Nyāya: one of the *Ṣaḍ-Darśana*, spiritual philosophies, which also include *Sāṅkhya*, *Mīmāṃsa*, *Vaiśeṣika*, *Yoga* and *Vedānta.*

Oestrogen: a hormone often referred to as a female hormone and relates to the menstrual cycle.

Ojas: our vitality and immunity. It's like nectar.

Ovulation phase: the time around the middle of the menstrual cycle when we ovulate.

Pañchakarma: specific *Āyurvedic* cleansing and detox treatments which include diet, herbs, treatments and massages. Traditionally a full four weeks of intense practices.

Pañcāmahābhūtas: the five great elements of earth, water, fire, air and space.

Pelvic floor: also known as the pelvic diaphragm. The muscles at the base of the pelvic bowl.

Pawanmuktāsana: known as the wind-releasing sequence from the Bihar School of yoga tradition. The one we refer to in this book relates to the abdomen.

Perimenopause: the time around menopause. Usually referring to any symptoms experienced in the time around menopause.

Pitta doṣa: the qualities of the fire and water elements. It is usually mostly associated with the heat of fire.

Prakṛti: the unique balanced combination of *doṣas* we had when we were conceived. Also the creative potential as seen in *Sāṅkhya* philosophy.

Prāṇa: often translated as the lifeforce energy. It is the vital force.

Prāṇa vāyu: the inhale, the 'forward moving breath'.

Prāṇayāma: the breathing practices associated with yoga and yoga classes.

Prasūti: obstetrics.

Pṛthvī: the element of earth also called *bhūmī*.

Progesterone: a hormone released from the ovaries. Often referred to as a chill-out and relaxing hormone.

Prostaglandins: hormone-like substances made on sites of injury. Prostaglandins are part of the healing process, which mean they can cause inflammation and pain.

Puruṣa: pure Consciousness and the Ultimate Truth. Formless and where it all begins.

Rajas: the *guna* of passion and activity.

Rakta dhātu: the blood tissue.

Raktamokṣa: bloodletting.

Rasāyana: the branch of *Āyurveda* dedicated to rejuvenation.

RED-S: relative energy deficiency in sport. When people expend more energy than they take in.

Ṣaḍ-Darśana: the philosophies of *Sāṅkhya*, *Nyāya*, *Vaiśeṣika*, *Mīmāṃsa*, *Yoga* and *Vedānta*.

Śakti: The creating force or Goddess. Also written as *Shakti*.

Sāmana vāyu: equalizing breath associated with the abdomen.

Sāṅkhya: the philosophy explained in Chapter 2 along with the enumeration and principles of the philosophy.

Sattva: quality of knowledge and bliss.

Shala: yoga studio or a home.

Śiva: Hindu God of life and destruction. Also written as Shiva.

Soma: plant or elixir of immortality. *Soma* is the nectar of contentment and bliss.

Strīroga: gynaecology.

Suśruta-saṃhitā: one of the classical *Āyurvedic* texts.

Tāmas: the quality, or guna, of ignorance and inertia.

Tāṇḍava: the divine dance of life and destruction danced by *Śiva*.

Tanmatra: the five sense perceptions: sound, touch, sight, taste and odour.

Tantra: a sacred path to liberation and ecstasy. Both Hinduism and Buddhism have esoteric paths of *tantric* wisdom. Please note *tantra* has nothing to do with the neo-*tantrik*, or 'new-age', association of sexual expression. Traditional *tantra* can be an embodied experience where practices for very advanced practitioners may include sexual ritual and pleasure. *Tantra* can also be translated as a method or technique such as *śālākyatantra* (surgery), one of *Āyurveda*'s eight branches of medicine.

Tejas: the pure fire and illumination of *pitta doṣa.*

Udāna vāyu: the upward moving flow of air.

Ujjâyî prāṇayāma: known as the ocean sound breath and the victorious breath. It creates a long slow breath with a sound in the throat.

Uterus: also called the womb. Part of the female reproductive anatomy.

Vāta doṣa: the qualities of air and space.

Vaidyas: medical practitioner.

Vaiśeṣika: one of the *Ṣaḍ-Darśana*, spiritual philosophies, which also include *Sāṅkhya, Mīmāṃsa, Nyāya, Yoga* and *Vedānta.*

Vāyu: the air or wind element.

Vedānta: one of the *Ṣaḍ-Darśana*, spiritual philosophies, which also include *Sāṅkhya, Mīmāṃsa, Nyāya, Yoga* and *Vaiśeṣika.*

Vedic/Vedas: Indian scriptures consisting of the *Rig Veda, Sama Veda, Yajur Veda*, and *Atharva Veda*. It is said that the wisdom from these sacred texts comes from the sages or Gods themselves.

Vinyāsa: means placing. In Western yoga, we refer to *vinyāsa* yoga as a practice where we are placing or moving our body in a specific way, usually in a flow-style yoga sequence connected with the breath.

Vkṛti: the current state of the *doṣas* and how they express themselves at this moment.

Vyāna vāyu: the all-pervading movement of *prāṇa.*

Womb: another word for uterus.

Vin yoga: a style of yoga where the poses are held for several minutes. A relaxing style of yoga often using plenty of props for support.

Yogāsana: yoga poses or postures, taught in most Western yoga classes.

Yoga nidra: literally yogīc sleep. A deep guided practise of various techniques to bring physical and mental relaxation.

Yogi Bhajan: see *kuṇḍalinī* yoga.

Yogīc: relating to yoga activity or philosophy.

Yoni: the female reproductive system – vulva, vagina, cervix, uterus, endometrium, ovaries and uterine tubes.

References

Classic *Āyurvedic* references

Āyurveda is a living science and art, and is built on three great classic texts (the *Bṛhat-Trayī*); *Caraka-saṃhitā*, *Suśruta-saṃhitā* and *Aṣṭāṅga-hṛdayam*. I have chosen not to cite every reference to the classic texts. Instead, I am sharing the volumes of the texts which I continuously study, and refer to in this book.

Caraka, Caraka Samhita Vol. I (2008) trans. R.K. Sharma & B. Dash. Varanasi: Chowkhamba Sanskrit Series Office.

Caraka, Caraka Samhita Vol. II–VI (2009) trans. R. K. Sharma & B. Dash. Varanasi: Chowkhamba Sanskrit Series Office.

Caraka, Caraka Samhita Vol. VII (2007) trans. R.K. Sharma & B. Dash. Varanasi: Chowkhamba Sanskrit Series Office.

Sushruta, The Sushruta Samhita: An English Translation Based on Original Sanskrit Text. Vol. 1–3 (2006) trans. K. Lal Bhishagratna. New Delhi: Cosmo Publications.

The *Ayurvediya Prasutitantra evam striroga* are not classical texts but rather excellent references to the classics in gynaecological knowledge.

Tiwari, P.V. (2009) *Ayurvediya Prasutitantra evam striroga, Part l Prasutitantra (obstetrics)*. Varanasi: Chaukhambha Orientalia.

Tiwari, P.V. (2009) *Ayurvediya Prasutitantra evam striroga, Part ll Striroga (gynecology)*. Varanasi: Chaukhambha Orientalia.

Vagbhata, Astanga Hrdayam Vol. 1 (2007) trans. Prof. K.R. Srikanth Murthy (fifth edition). Varanasi: Chowkharmba Krishnas Academy.

Vagbhata, Astanga Hrdayam Vol. 2–3 (2008) trans. Prof. K.R. Srikanth Murthy (fifth edition). Varanasi: Chowkharmba Krishnas Academy.

Introduction

Bachman, N. (2005) *The Language of Yoga*. Louisville, CO: Sounds True.

Bachman, N. (2006) *The Language of Āyurveda*. Victoria, BC, Canada: Trafford Publishing.

Soumpasis, I., Grace, B. & Johnson, S. (2020) Real-life insights on menstrual cycles and ovulation using big data. *Human Reproduction Open*, 2. doi: 10.1093/hropen/hoaa011.

Wisdom Library, www.wisdomlib.org, accessed throughout the writing period.

Chapter 1: Yoga and the Menstrual Cycle

Ashtanga Yoga Austin. Lady's holidays, https://ashtangayogaaustin.com/ladys-holiday, accessed 7 Dec 2021.

Cartwright, T., Mason, H., Porter, A. & Pilkington, K. (2020) Yoga practice in the UK: A cross-sectional survey of motivation, health benefits and behaviours. *BMJ Open*, doi: 10.e031848.10.1136/bmjopen-2019-031848.

Cramer, H., Ward, L., Steel, A., Lauche, R., Dobos, G. & Zhang, Y. (2016) Prevalence, patterns, and predictors of yoga use: Results of a U.S. Nationally Representative Survey. *American Journal of Preventative Medicine*, 50(2), 230–235. doi: 10.1016/j.amepre.2015.07.037.

Criado Perez, C. (2019) *Invisible Women*. London: Vintage.

Iyengar, B.K.S. (1991) *Light on Yoga*. India: Harper Collins.

KYM. Krishnamacharya Yoga Mandiram, www.kym.org/about-kym, accessed 7 Dec 2021.

Liu, K.A. & Mager, N.A. (2016) Women's involvement in clinical trials: Historical perspective and future implications. *Pharmacy Practice*, 14(1), 708. https://doi.org/10.18549/PharmPract.2016.01.708.

Moon days, Astanga Yoga London. Moon days, www.astangayogalondon.com/moon-days, accessed 7 Dec 2021.

Ravindran, T.S., Teerawattananon, Y., Tannenbaum, C. & Vijayasingham, L. (2020). Making pharmaceutical research and regulation work for women. *British Medical Journal*, 371, m3808. doi:10.1136/bmj.m3808.

Saraswati, S.S. (1996) *Asana Pranayama Mudra Bandha*, India: Yoga Publications Trust.

Swami Sivananda. Divine Life Society, www.sivanandaonline.org/?cmd=displaysection&section_id=1645&parent=1055&format=html, accessed 7 Dec 2021.

Tirumalai Krishnamacharya, Wikipedia, https://en.wikipedia.org/wiki/Tirumalai_Krishnamacharya, accessed 7 Dec 2021.

Veronesi, U., Luini, A., Mariani, L., Del Vecchio, M. *et al.* (1994) Effect of menstrual phase on surgical treatment of breast cancer. *The Lancet*, 343(8912), 1545–1547. https://doi.org/10.1016/S0140-6736(94)92942-4.

Woitowich, N.C., Beery, A. & Woodruff, T. (2020) A 10-year follow-up study of sex inclusion in the biological sciences. *eLife*, 9, e56344. https://doi.org/10.7554/eLife.56344.

Yoga Journal and Yoga Alliance (2016) *The 2016 Yoga in America Study*. www.yogaalliance.org/Portals/0/2016%20Yoga%20in%20America%20Study%20RESULTS.pdf, accessed 7 Dec 2021.

Chapter 2: *Sāṅkhya* Philosophy

Frawley, D. (2004) *Ayurveda and the Mind*. Delhi: Motilal Banarsidass.

Lad, V. (2002) *Textbook of Ayurveda Fundamental Principles*. Albuquerque, NM: The Ayurvedic Press.

Chapter 3: Understanding *Āyurveda* and the *Doṣas*

Dick, M. (2021) The Ancient Ayurvedic Writings, www.ayurveda.com/the-ancient-ayurvedic-writings, accessed 16 Nov 2021.

Loukas, M., Lanteri, A., Ferrauiola, J., Tubbs, R.S. *et al.* (2010) Anatomy in ancient India: A focus on the Susruta Samhita. *Journal of Anatomy*, 217, 646–650. https://doi.org/10.1111/j.1469-7580.2010.01294.x.

Chapter 4: The *Āyurvedic* and Cultural View of the Menstrual Cycle

ACOG Committee Opinion No. 651: Menstruation in girls and adolescents: Using the menstrual cycle as a vital sign. (2015) *Obstetrics and Gynecology*, 126(6), e143–e146. doi:10.1097/AOG.0000000000001215.

Joseph, S. (2020) *Rtu Vidya*. Tamil Nadu: Notion Press.

Kokkoka, P. (1965) *Ratishastra*, trans. S.C. Upadhyaya. Bombay: D.B. Taraporevala.

Letters, Notes, and Answers to Correspondents. (1878) *British Medical Journal*, 1(902), 553–554.

Sridhar, N. (2019) *Menstruation Across Cultures*. New Delhi: Vistasta Publishing.

Yoni Tantra (1995) trans. M. Magee. Harrow: Worldwide Tantra Series.

Chapter 5: Lunar Flow and Connecting with the Moon

Mayatitananda (2007) *Women's Power to Heal Through Inner Medicine*. Washington, DC: Mother Om Media.

Chapter 7: Western Physiology and Hormones

Agoulnik, A.I. (2007) Relaxin and related peptides in male reproduction. *Advances in Experimental Medicine and Biology*, 612, 49–64. https://doi.org/10.1007/978-0-387-74672-2_5.

Hansen, A., Vendelbo Jensen, D., Larsen, E., Wilken-Jensen, C. & Kjeld Petersen, L. (1996) Relaxin is not related to symptom-giving pelvic girdle relaxation in pregnant women. *Acta Obstetricia et Gynecologica Scandinavica*, 75(3), 245–249. doi: 10.3109/00016349609047095.

Miller, G., Tybur, J. & Jordan, B. (2007) Ovulatory cycle effects on tip earnings by lap dancers: Economic evidence for human estrus? *Evolution and Human Behavior*, 28(6), 375–381. https://doi.org/10.1016/j.evolhumbehav.2007.06.002.

Petersen, L.K., Hvidman, L. & Uldbjerg, N. (1994) Normal serum relaxin in women with disabling pelvic pain during pregnancy. *Gynecologic and Obsterict Investigation*, 38(1), 21–23. doi: 10.1159/000292438.

Romero-Moraleda, B., Coso, J.D., Gutiérrez-Hellín, J., Ruiz-Moreno, C., Grgic, J. & Lara, B. (2019) The influence of the menstrual cycle on muscle strength and power performance. *Journal of Human Kinetics*, 68(1), 123–133. https://doi.org/10.2478/hukin-2019-0061.

Soumpasis, I., Grace, B. & Johnson, S. (2020) Real-life insights on menstrual cycles and ovulation using big data. *Human Reproduction Open*, 2. doi: 10.1093/hropen/hoaa011.

Wojtys, E.M., Huston, L.J., Lindenfeld, T.N., Hewett, T.E. & Greenfield, M.L.V.H. (1998) Association between the menstrual cycle and anterior cruciate ligament injuries in female athletes. *American Journal of Sports Medicine*, 26(5), 614–619. doi: 10.1177/03635465980260050301.

Wreje, U., Kristiansson, P., Aberg, H., Byström, B. & von Schoultz, B. (1995) Serum levels of relaxin during the menstrual cycle and oral contraceptive use. *Gynecologic and Obstetric Investigation*, 39(3), 197–200. https://doi.org/10.1159/000292408.

Wu, W.L., Lin, T.Y., Chu, I.H. & Liang, J.M. (2015) The acute effects of yoga on cognitive measures for women with premenstrual syndrome. *Journal of Alternative and Complementary Medicine*, 21(6), 364–369. https://doi.org/10.1089/acm.2015.0070.

Chapter 8: *Āyurvedic* Physiology and the Menstrual Phases

Lad, V. (2002) *Textbook of Ayurveda Fundamental Principles*. Albuquerque, NM: The Ayurvedic Press.

Chapter 9: From Menarche to Menopause

Elavsky, S. & McAuley, E. (2007) Physical activity and mental health outcomes during menopause: A randomized controlled trial. *Annals of Behavioral Medicine*, 33(2), 132–142. https://doi.org/10.1007/BF02879894.

Jorge, M.P., Santaella, D.F., Pontes, I.M.O., Shiramizu, V.K.M. *et al.* (2016) Hatha Yoga practice decreases menopause symptoms and improves quality of life: A randomized controlled trial. *Complementary Therapies in Medicine*, 26: 128–135. https://doi.org/10.1016/j.ctim.2016.03.014.

Mayatitananda (2007) *Women's Power to Heal Through Inner Medicine*. Washington, DC: Mother Om Media.

National Health Service (2018) *Overview menopause*, www.nhs.uk/conditions/menopause, accessed 7 Aug 2021.

Pope, A. & Wurlitzer, H. (2017) *Wild Power* (first edition). London: Hay House.

van Driel, C.M., Stuursma, A., Schroevers, M.J., Mourits, M.J. & de Bock, G.H. (2019) Mindfulness, cognitive behavioural and behaviour-based therapy for natural and treatment-induced menopausal symptoms: A systematic review and meta-analysis. *BJOG*, 126(3), 330–339. doi: 10.1111/1471-0528.15153

Wong, C., Yip, B.H.K., Gao, T. *et al.* (2018) Mindfulness-based stress reduction (MBSR) or psychoeducation for the reduction of menopausal symptoms: A randomized, controlled clinical trial. *Scientific Reports*, 8, 6609. https://doi.org/10.1038/s41598-018-24945-4.

Chapter 10: Bringing it All Together: Yoga, *Āyurveda*, Hormones and the Menstrual Cycle

Costello, J.T., Bieuzen, F. & Bleakley, C.M. (2014) Where are all the female participants in sports and exercise medicine research? *European Journal of Sports Science*, 14(8), 847–851. doi: 10.1080/17461391.2014.911354.

Cowley, E.S., Olenick, A.A., McNulty, K.L. & Ross, E.Z. (2021) 'Invisible sportswomen': The sex data gap in sport and exercise science research. *Women in Sport and Physical Activity Journal*, 29(2), 1–6. doi.org/10.1123/wspaj.2021-0028.

McNulty, K.L., Elliott-Sale, K.J., Dolan, E. *et al.* (2020) The effects of menstrual cycle phase on exercise performance in eumenorrheic women: A systematic review and meta-analysis. *Sports Medicine*, 50, 1813–1827. https://doi.org/10.1007/s40279-020-01319-3.

Steinberg, J.R., Turner, B.E., Weeks, B.T. *et al.* (2021) Analysis of female enrollment and participant sex by burden of disease in US clinical trials between 2000 and 2020. *JAMA Network Open*, 4(6), e2113749. doi:10.1001/jamanetworkopen.2021.13749.

Chapter 11: Practical Application of *Āyurvedic* Principles in Yoga

Lange, A. (2009) *A critical literature review of the evidence for yoga asana's effect on mental health*. BSc Complementary Health Sciences (Ayurveda), Middlesex University, London.

Mind (2020) *Mental health facts and statistics*, www.mind.org.uk/information-support/types-of-mental-health-problems/statistics-and-facts-about-mental-health/how-common-are-mental-health-problems, accessed 4 Aug 2021.

National Health Service (2019) *Overview obesity*, www.nhs.uk/conditions/obesity, accessed 4 Aug 2021.

Chapter 12: Yoga for Each Phase of the Menstrual Cycle

Agoulnik, A.I. (2007) Relaxin and related peptides in male reproduction. *Advances in Experimental Medicine and Biology*, 612, 49–64. https://doi.org/10.1007/978-0-387-74672-2_5.

Bayer, U. & Hausmann, M. (2012) Menstrual cycle-related changes of functional cerebral asymmetries in fine motor coordination. *Brain and Cognition*, 79(1), 34–38.

Beynnon, B.D. & Shultz, S.J. (2008) Anatomic alignment, menstrual cycle phase, and the risk of anterior cruciate ligament injury. *Journal of Athletic Training*, 43(5), 541–542. https://doi.org/10.4085/1062-6050-43.5.541.

Fridén, C., Hirschberg, A.L., Saartok, T. & Renström, P. (2006) Knee joint kinaesthesia and neuromuscular coordination during three phases of the menstrual cycle in moderately active women. Knee surgery, sports traumatology, arthroscopy. *Official Journal of the ESSKA*, 14(4), 383–389. https://doi.org/10.1007/s00167-005-0663-4.

Ghati, N., Killa, A.K., Sharma, G., Karunakaran, B. *et al.* (2021) A randomized trial of the immediate effect of Bee-Humming Breathing exercise on blood pressure and heart rate variability in patients with essential hypertension. *Explore*, 17(4), 312–319. https://doi.org/10.1016/j.explore.2020.03.009.

Hansen, A., Jensen, D.V., Larsen, E., Wilken-Jensen, C. & Petersen, L.K. (1996) Relaxin is not related to symptom-giving pelvic girdle relaxation in pregnant women. *Acta Obstetricia et Gynecologica Scandinavica*, 75(3), 245–249. https://doi.org/10.3109/00016349609047095.

Herzberg, S.D., Motu'apuaka, M.L., Lambert, W., Fu, R., Brady, J. & Guise, J.M. (2017) The effect of menstrual cycle and contraceptives on ACL injuries and laxity: A systematic review and meta-analysis. *Orthopaedic Journal of Sports Medicine*, 5(7). https://doi.org/10.1177/2325967117718781.

Iyengar, B.K.S. (1991) *Light on Yoga*. India: Harper Collins.

Knowles, O.E., Aisbett, B., Main, L.C., Drinkwater, E.J., Orellana, L. & Lamon, S. (2019) Resistance training and skeletal muscle protein metabolism in eumenorrheic females: Implications for researchers and practitioners. *Sports Medicine*, 49(11), 1637–1650.

Martin, D., Timmins, K., Cowie, C., Alty, J. *et al.* (2021) Injury incidence across the menstrual cycle in international footballers. *Frontiers in Sports and Active Living*, 3, 616999. https://doi.org/10.3389/fspor.2021.616999.

Melegario, S., Simão, R., Vale, R., Batista, L. & Novaes, J. (2006) The influence of the menstrual cycle on the flexibility in practitioners of gymnastics at fitness centers. *Revista Brasileira de Medicina do Esporte*, 12, 125–128.

Miller, G., Tybur, J. & Jordan, B. (2007) Ovulatory cycle effects on tip earnings by lap dancers: Economic evidence for human estrus? *Evolution and Human Behavior*, 28(6), 375–381.

Miyazaki, M. & Maeda, S. (2022) Changes in hamstring flexibility and muscle strength during the menstrual cycle in healthy young females. *Journal of Physical Therapy Science*, 34(2), 92–98.

Myklebust, G., Mæhlum, S., Holm, I. & Bahr, R. (1998) A prospective cohort study of anterior cruciate ligament injuries in elite Norwegian team handball. *Scandinavian Journal of Medicine & Science in Sports*, 8, 149–153. https://doi.org/10.1111/j.1600-0838.1998.tb00185.x.

National Health Service (2020) *Exercise in pregnancy*, www.nhs.uk/pregnancy/keeping-well/exercise, accessed 14 Aug 2021.

Oosthuyse, T. & Bosch, A.N. (2010) The effect of the menstrual cycle on exercise metabolism: Implications for exercise performance in eumenorrhoeic women. *Sports Medicine*, 40(3), 207–227. doi: 10.2165/11317090-000000000-00000.

Petersen, L.K., Hvidman, L. & Uldbjerg, N. (1994) Normal serum relaxin in women with disabling pelvic pain during pregnancy. *Gynecologic and Obstetric Investigation*, 38(1), 21–23. https://doi.org/10.1159/000292438.

Rakhshaee, Z. (2011) Effect of three yoga poses (cobra, cat and fish poses) in women with primary dysmenorrhea: A randomized clinical trial. *Journal of Pediatric and Adolescent Gynecology*, 24(4), 192–196. https://doi.org/10.1016/j.jpag.2011.01.059.

Saraswati, S.S. (1996) *Āsana Prāṇayāma Mudrā Bandha*. India: Yoga Publications Trust.

Wojtys, E.M., Huston, L.J., Lindenfeld, T.N., Hewett, T.E. & Greenfield, M.L. (1998) Association between the menstrual cycle and anterior cruciate ligament injuries in female athletes. *American Journal of Sports Medicine*, 26(5), 614–619. https://doi.org/10.1177/036354659 80260050301.

Wreje, U., Kristiansson, P., Aberg, H., Byström, B. & von Schoultz, B. (1995) Serum levels of relaxin during the menstrual cycle and oral contraceptive use. *Gynecologic and Obstetric Investigation*, 39(3), 197–200. https://doi.org/10.1159/000292408.

Wu, W.L., Lin, T.Y., Chu, I.H. & Liang, J.M. (2015) The acute effects of yoga on cognitive measures for women with premenstrual syndrome. *Journal of Alternative and Complementary Medicine*, 21(6), 364–369. https://doi.org/10.1089/acm.2015.0070.

Chapter 13: Rest, Relaxation and Rejuvenation

Frawley, D. (2012) *Soma in Yoga and Ayurveda*. Twin Lakes, WI: Lotus Press.

Lad, V. (2002) *Textbook of Ayurveda Fundamental Principles*. Albuquerque, NM: The Ayurvedic Press.

National Health Service (2018) *Overview – Generalised anxiety disorder in adults*, www.nhs.uk/mental-health/conditions/generalised-anxiety-disorder/overview, accessed 27 Sept 2021.

Chapter 14: Yoga for Specific Complaints

Ansari R.M. (2016) Kapalabhati pranayama: An answer to modern day polycystic ovarian syndrome and coexisting metabolic syndrome? *International Journal of Yoga*, 9(2), 163–167. https://doi.org/10.4103/0973-6131.183705.

Broderick, A., Kennedy, S. & Zondervan, K. (2013) Epidemiology of Chronic Pelvic Pain. In G.F. Gebhart, & R.F. Schmidt (eds) *Encyclopedia of Pain*. Berlin, Heidelberg: Springer.

Bustan, M.N., Seweng, A. & Ernawati (2018) Abdominal stretching exercise in decreasing pain of dysmenorrhea among nursing students. *Journal of Physics: Conference Series*, 1028(1). doi: 10.1088/1742-6596/1028/1/012103.

Dayani Siriwardene, S.A., Karunathilaka, L.P., Kodituwakku, N.D. & Karunarathne, Y.A. (2010) Clinical efficacy of Ayurveda treatment regimen on subfertility with polycystic ovarian syndrome (PCOS). *Ayu*, 31(1), 24–27. https://doi.org/10.4103/0974-8520.68203.

Dhiman, K. (2014) Ayurvedic intervention in the management of uterine fibroids: A case series. *Ayu, 35*(3), 303–308. https://doi.org/10.4103/0974-8520.153750.

Gonçalves, A.V., Barros, N.F. & Bahamondes, L. (2017) The practice of hatha yoga for the treatment of pain associated with endometriosis. *Journal of Alternative and Complementary Medicine*, 23(1). http://doi.org/10.1089/acm.2015.0343.

Gonçalves, A.V., Makuch, M.Y., Setubal, M.S., Barros, N.F. & Bahamondes, L. (2016) A qualitative study on the practice of yoga for women with pain-associated endometriosis. *Journal of Alternative and Complementary Medicine*, 22(12), 977–982. https://doi.org/10.1089/acm.2016.0021.

Hall, E. & Steiner, M. (2013) Serotonin and female psychopathology. *Women's Health*, 85–97. https://doi.org/10.2217/WHE.12.64.

Jadhao, V.S. (2019) Impact of yoga training intervention on menstrual disorders. *International Journal of Physiology, Nutrition and Physical Education*, 4(1), 1147–1149.

Kadam, R., Shinde, K., Kadam, R. & Kulkarni, M.S. (2014) Contemporary and traditional perspectives of polycystic ovarian syndrome (PCOS): A critical review. *IOSR Journal of Dental and Medical Sciences*, 13(9), 89–98.

Kumaravelu, P. & Das, D.K. (2020) Effect of yogic practices on selected hematological variable among college girls suffering with irregular menstruation. *Mukt Shabd Journal*, 9(8), 1761–1765.

Lin, Y.H., Chen, Y.H., Chang, H.Y., Au, H.K., Tzeng, C.R. & Huang, Y.H. (2018) Chronic niche inflammation in endometriosis-associated infertility: Current understanding and future therapeutic strategies. *International Journal of Molecular Sciences*, 19(8), 2385. https://doi.org/10.3390/ijms19082385.

Mohseni, M., Eghbali, M., Bahrami, H., Dastaran, F. & Amini, L. (2021) Yoga effects on anthropometric indices and polycystic ovary syndrome symptoms in women undergoing infertility treatment: A randomized controlled clinical trial. *Evidence-Based Complementary and Alternative Medicine*, eCAM, 2021, 5564824. https://doi.org/10.1155/2021/5564824.

Monika, R., Singh, U., Ghildiyal, A., Kala, S. & Srivastava, N. (2012) Effect of yoga nidra on physiological variables in patients of menstrual disturbances of reproductive age group. *Indian Journal of Physiology and Pharmacology*, 56(2), 161–167.

Motahari-Tabari, N., Shirvani, M.A. & Alipour, A. (2017) Comparison of the effect of stretching exercises and mefenamic acid on the reduction of pain and menstruation characteristics in primary dysmenorrhea: A randomized clinical trial. *Oman Medical Journal*, 32(1), 47–53. https://doi.org/10.5001/omj.2017.09.

National Health and Medical Research Council (2018) International evidence based guideline for the assessment and management of polycystic ovary syndrome. Monash University, Melbourne Australia, https://www.monash.edu/__data/assets/pdf_file/0004/1412644/PCOS_Evidence-Based-Guidelines_20181009.pdf, accessed 22 Aug 2022.

National Health Service (2018) *Overview fibroids*, www.nhs.uk/conditions/fibroids, accessed 4 Oct 2021.

National Health Service (2019) *Ovulation pain*, www.nhs.uk/conditions/ovulation-pain, accessed 17 Oct 2021.

National Health Service (2021) *Premenstrual syndrome (PMS)*, www.nhs.uk/conditions/pre-menstrual-syndrome, accessed 18 Oct 2021.

National Health Service (2021a) *Overview heavy periods*, www.nhs.uk/conditions/heavy-periods, accessed 5 Nov 2021.

National Health Service (2021b) *Irregular periods*, www.nhs.uk/conditions/irregular-periods, accessed 5 Nov 2021.

National Institute for Health and Care Excellence (2020), *Amenorrhoea*, https://cks.nice.org.uk/topics/amenorrhoea, accessed 5 Nov 2021.

Nidhi, R., Padmalatha, V., Nagarathna, R. & Amritanshu, R. (2012) Effect of holistic yoga program on anxiety symptoms in adolescent girls with polycystic ovarian syndrome: A randomized control trial. *International Journal of Yoga*, 5(2), 112–117. https://doi.org/10.4103/0973-6131.98223.

Patel, V., Menezes, H., Menezes, C., Bouwer, S., Bostick-Smith, C.A. & Speelman, D.L. (2020) Regular mindful yoga practice as a method to improve androgen levels in women with polycystic ovary syndrome: A randomized, controlled trial. *Journal of the American Osteopathic Association*. https://doi.org/10.7556/jaoa.2020.050.

Rakhshaee, Z. (2011) Effect of three yoga poses (cobra, cat and fish poses) in women with primary dysmenorrhea: A randomized clinical trial. *Journal of Pediatric and Adolescent Gynecology*, 24(4), 192–196. https://doi.org/10.1016/j.jpag.2011.01.059.

Rejeki, S., Yuliani Pratama, F., Ernawati, E., Yanto, A., Soesanto, E. & Pranata, S. (2021) Abdominal stretching as a therapy for dysmenorrhea. *Open Access Macedonian Journal of Medical Sciences*, 9(G), 180–183.

Rosyida, D. & Suwandono, A., Ariyanti, I., Suhartono, D., Mashoedi, I.F. & Fatmasari, D. (2017) Comparison of effect of abdominal stretching exercise and pain intensity in teenage girls. *Belitung Nursing Journal*, 3(3), 221–228.

Russell, N., Daniels, B., Smoot, B. & Allen, D. (2019) Effects of yoga on quality of life and pain in women with chronic pelvic pain: Systematic review and meta-analysis. *Journal of Women's Health Physical Therapy*, 43(3), 144–154. doi: 10.1097/JWH.0000000000000135.

Satyanand, V., Hymavathi, K., Panneerselvam, E., Mahaboobvali, S., Basha, S.A. & Shoba, C. (2014) Effects of yogasanas in the management of pain during menstruation. *Journal of Medical Science and Scientific Research*, 2(11), 2969–2974.

Stachenfeld, N.S. (2008) Sex hormone effects on body fluid regulation. *Exercise and Sport Sciences Reviews*, 36(3), 152–159. https://doi.org/10.1097/JES.0b013e31817be928.

Vanitha, A., Pandiaraja, M., Maheshkumar, K. & Venkateswaran, S.T. (2018) Effect of yoga nidra on resting cardiovascular parameters in polycystic ovarian syndrome women. *National Journal of Physiology, Pharmacy and Pharmacology*, 8(11), 1505–1508. doi:10.5455/njppp.2018.8.0411112082018.

Chapter 16: Perimenopause Leading to Change

National Health Service (2018) *Symptoms menopause*, www.nhs.uk/conditions/menopause/symptoms, accessed 10 Nov 2021.

Willacy, H. (2021) *Progestogen-only contraceptive pill*. Patient. https://patient.info/sexual-health/hormone-pills-patches-and-rings/progestogen-only-contraceptive-pill-pop, accessed 4 May 2022.

Index